Home ♥ Made Health

Also by Raymond and Dorothy Moore

Home-Spun Schools
Home-Grown Kids
Home-Style Teaching
Better Late than Early
School Can Wait

Home ♥ Made Health

A Family Guide to Nutrition, Exercise, Stress Control, and Preventive Medicine

Raymond & Dorothy Moore

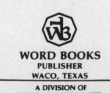

WORD BOOKS
PUBLISHER
WACO, TEXAS

A DIVISION OF
WORD, INCORPORATED

HOMEMADE HEALTH

Copyright © 1986 by Raymond and Dorothy Moore

Unless otherwise specified, all scripture quotations are from the Authorized King James Version. Those marked NIV are from the New International Version, © 1978 by the New York International Bible Society, used by permission of Zondervan Bible Publishers. Those marked LB are from *The Living Bible*, © 1971 by Tyndale House Publishers, and are used by permission

Library of Congress Cataloguing-in-Publication Data

Moore, Dorothy N.
  Homemade health.

  1. Family—Health and hygiene. 2. Nutrition.
3. Health. 4. Christian life—1960–
I. Moore, Raymond S. II. Title. [DNLM: 1. Alternative
Medicine—popular works. WB 130 M821h]
RA777.7M66 1986   613   86–15874
ISBN 0–8499–0606–7

67898 BKC 987654321

Printed in the United States of America

To a godly physician,
    Marion Barnard, M.D.,
and his wife, Cleo:
        and
    to a great Christian dentist,
    James Dutro, D.D.S.,
    and his wife, Joyce.
and to the distinguished medical and
    scientific board who gave this book a
    credibility uncommon to health books today.

Contents

A Fence or an Ambulance

'Twas a dangerous cliff, as they freely confessed,
Though to walk near its crest was so pleasant;
But over its terrible edge there had slipped
A duke and full many a peasant.
So the people said something would have to be done,
But their projects did not at all tally;
Some said, "Put a fence around the edge of the cliff,"
Some, "An ambulance down in the valley."
But the cry for the ambulance carried the day,
For it spread through the neighboring city;
A fence may be useful or not, it is true,
But each heart became brimful of pity
For those who slipped over that dangerous cliff;
And the dwellers in highway and alley
Gave pounds or gave pence not to put up a fence,
But an ambulance down in the valley.

"For the cliff is all right, if you're careful," they said,
"And, if folks even slip and are dropping,
It isn't the slipping that hurts them so much,
As the shock down below when they're stopping."
So day after day, as these mishaps occurred,
Quick forth would these rescuers sally
To pick up the victims who fell off the cliff,
With their ambulance down in the valley.
Then an old sage remarked: "It's a marvel to me
That people give far more attention
To repairing results than to stopping the cause,
When they'd much better aim at prevention.
Let us stop at its source all this mischief," cried he,
"Come, neighbors and friends, let us rally;
If the cliff we will fence we might almost dispense
With the ambulance down in the valley."

JOSEPH MALINS

Professional Advisory Panel

Beloved, I wish above all things that
thou mayest prosper and be in health,
even as thy soul prospereth.

3 John 2

Prologue

While we cannot honestly apologize for the principles in this book, we do beg your forgiveness if or when we offend. We have tried to avoid offense while candidly telling a well-documented story that needs to be told. And we urge you to make any changes you believe best for you, patiently and with deliberation. *We do not urge you to rush into every reform suggested in this book.* Some may not be for you. Check out the evidence, counsel with your physician if necessary, and take your time.

This book is not for faddists. It is intended for those who genuinely seek the best for their families and themselves. It is not a medical bible or handbook intended to displace your physician. God has given these men and women to us, just as Christ called the physician Luke. There is no greater human exemplar of the mission of Christ than a qualified physician who genuinely ministers. It has been our purpose to bring together the findings of top physicians and scientists, under the scrutiny of a panel of highly successful research and practicing professionals in such specialty fields as allergy, cardiology, dentistry, epidemiology, general practice, health education, immunology, internal medicine, neurology, OB-Gyn, ophthalmology, otology, pediatrics, psychiatry, public health, several surgical specialties, and veterinary medicine. We have included an indepth addendum on osteoporosis and the current calcium scare because of its timeliness in relation to the total message of this book. Yet none of the members of our physician–dentist–veterinarian panel are responsible in any way for the statements made in this book. Nor are we at all sure that all on the panel agree with all others in all things; this might be unfortunate.

Dorothy and I accept total responsibility for the direction and suggestions in this book. She worked at least as hard as I. She is *at least* equal as author. We mutually decided to write it in first person, since on several occasions we needed to refer to her. And because of her modest but thorough experience in health and nutrition over the past fifty years, and her recent unique experience in remedy, this book has perhaps even more meaning to her.

Finally, we ask you to remember this: We have written in the certainty that all our health habits contribute to our characters and those of our families. They either build up or tear down our bodies and our brains—the organs which function as your mind and mine, the seat of our conscience, the center of our communication with God. It is our prayer and hope that you may prosper in body and soul as you prepare for an eternity with your Maker, *and live as preparing to step into heaven at the soon coming of the King.*

—RAYMOND S. MOORE

Home ♥ Made Health

Whether . . . ye eat, or drink, or whatsoever ye do, do all to the glory of
God.

1 Corinthians 10:31

1

Eat, Drink and Be Blessed

During our college days, veteran psychologist Guy Wolfkill often raised his index finger in a solemn admonition which came to make a lot of common sense to us. "If you want to live the fullest life for the longest time," Dr. Wolfkill warned, "you must learn to *sacrifice present pleasures for future benefits.*" Sounds simple, doesn't it? But it isn't, at all. In fact, your daily habits are almost sacred to you, and your appetite is usually the most sacred of all.

Said less cleverly: If you are determined to have a genuinely happy life, you must pay the price. It is not expensive in dollars, but it is in sense. It comes only by self-control, not by luck or special blessing, except as you may have long-lived ancestors whose heritage of health may give you some advantage. And the better an ancestor you are—if you can look ahead that far—the more grateful your descendants will be for their heritage of health.

Try an experiment with us as you read this chapter, and perhaps this book: Check your wisdom—your reasoning power—against the instincts of a mouse, a rat, or a dog. The mouse, remember, can reason but little. Like any animal except humans, he depends more upon instinct. Humans, the superior race, are given power to reason things out. Given the choice between white or whole wheat bread, oiled or natural nuts, white or brown rice, the average mouse or rat will invariably take the latter. Few animals will eat

13

to gain more weight than is best for them—unless, that is, they are domesticated by man (like fat cats and dogs). As you read, see how you react to the scientific and clinical evidence in this book. How do you choose?

Prisoner's Food

Our Western influence has been so pervasive in diet that top specialists in the Orient hold us accountable for introducing white rice, the staple today of the oriental diet. The peer pressure of the West was so powerful during World War II that brown rice—which most Japanese were forced to eat for economy's sake, was disdained as "prisoners' food." Even though Japanese nutritionists and physiologists noted the astonishingly taller growth of their youngsters of the War generation, the appeal of the West and their latent appetites for junk food recaptured the food market and still reigns today. Such is the appetite of man.

If we don't take time to be well, we'll have to take time to be sick. Sound health is a gift few of us appreciate until we lose it. And for many that is too late. Yet the highest and best development of our physical, mental, spiritual and social powers largely depends upon our health. Good health is as crucial for making happy parents and children as they are for making a happy home. This is why we set out to give you some principled health hints as the most recent volume in our series on happiness and fulfillment in the home.

God always sets before us an ideal—a star to reach for, a goal to seek. And His fondest wish for us is that we will allow Him to help restore in us His image which was lost in Eden—godliness, godlikeness. In the same way we are presenting to you an ideal which is fashioned according to the best of biblical and scientific data available to us along with our experiences in seeking to reach this goal. We have learned much in the last ten years and even more in the last five—and we are still in the process of implementing the things we know. The first two chapters present a crucial setting for lifestyle examination. If for some reason you can't bear this "preaching," please move on to Chapter 3.

Magic Pill?

Wouldn't it be great if science could discover a magic pill which would bring health to everyone! Or would it? We agree that our society would be in a much worse situation than it is if scientific discoveries had not added twenty years to our lives.

Yet medical science is baffled by new diseases it can neither explain nor cure. And it has made more than a few errors: drugs which have backfired with serious side effects and treatments which have killed more than cured. Would you welcome insights on some fundamentals of health which were given to man a long time ago, not only to remedy disease, but also to *prevent* it—and early death?

Suppose you find that you can stop the knock in your car's motor by either reducing its compression or buying a higher octane gasoline instead of your current brand. Which would you choose? Perhaps you decide against reducing compression because you need all the power you can get to climb those hills on the way home and to pass on that two-lane highway, and besides you find compression-reduction expense too high. Your mechanic also advises against reducing compression, yet suggests that you do something soon or you might irreparably damage your engine. In which event, of course, you *could* trade in your car for a new one!

So you decide to buy the better brand of gasoline—which also is cheaper and gives better mileage. But the service station is five miles down the road, and your present station attendant is an elder in your church (There go the peer pressures!). His youngsters are pals with your boys (There they go again!). And, woe is you, his wife is your darling's best friend! What do you do?

This is exactly where most of us are in coping with our bodies' demands—except that we can't trade for a new one if this one breaks down. It is a risk even to order a new *part* for your body!

Evidence of Maturity

Just how mature are you? Do you value truth? Are you determined to find it? And then to accept and live by it decisively regardless of its inconvenience or the risk your friends and neighbors might think you are a little strange? There are hundreds of health theory books, but few that are willing to face frankly the destructive lifestyles which pervade Western society today. These we seem to dearly cherish—or else we have become dangerously addicted to them.

We have set out to bring you solid scientific facts based on biblical principles which have been proven in the lives of thousands with the hope that you will recognize in these a way of life to *prevent* disease and be a blessing to all. There are divine reasons for every sound health habit. These are built into every cell of our bodies and govern every activity of our lives—including exercise, attitude and mental health, breathing, cleanliness, diet, dress, elimination, liquids, rest, recreation, recuperation, regularity, relaxation, sunshine, temperance and balance, and ultimate faith. God operates by principle and in an orderly way. He did not "experiment" when He planned the human body and He gave you and me principles which are absolutely fundamental.

Living by Principle

But again, when you live by principle you always find that there is a price to pay. Some simply are not that interested in future benefits. One dear Christian friend of ours clings to her cigarettes as if she will never have to meet her future. She insists that Christ will somehow "relieve" her of her problem "at an appropriate time." Another valued colleague with a family history of heart disease, candidly and honestly admits, "I like my lifestyle," even though in fact his is more of a "death style." We have neither chided nor quarreled with either of these unique people, yet what they are saying and acting out is, "My mind is made up; don't confuse me with facts."

One of our physician friends tells of a technique she sometimes uses and which more physicians might try: One of her patients had a series of distressing symptoms whose causes were well within his ability to cure. Instead of suggesting remedies, she wrote her patient's name on her prescription pad and began making notes while asking him what he would do if he were the doctor. After gentle urging, he hesitatingly suggested some solutions—e.g., less coffee and red meats, more exercise, more sleep, and no alcohol. These the doctor faithfully recorded on the prescription blank, signed her name, and handed it to him—an excellent self-prescribed program to solve his own problems.

Those Good Doctors

We strongly support the role of able, licensed physicians. Unfortunately, many of them are not well informed nutritionally and do not know how to prescribe the makings of a sound lifestyle. On the other hand, many worthy doctors are informed and vow that 90 percent of our ailments would go away if we simply did what we know we should do. Yet somehow we do not do what we know we should do. We pass off this advice, preferring immediate solutions over those which require lifestyle change. We hope that "a good night's rest" helped along by a sleeping pill and a couple of aspirin will take care of the situation—*now!*

Many otherwise honest doctors are certain that in order for their practices to survive they must give most people a "quick fix." They know that we don't want to face the consequences of our actions. *We will do it for our cars and our pets, but not for our bodies.*

Most of us have better sense than to challenge the law of gravity, because if we jump from a cliff, we know that the results will be immediate disaster. But since there is in most cases a delay in the natural laws of our bodies, it is easy for us to think, *Never mind, it won't happen to me.* Then when we least expect it, and perhaps when we are living our lives to the fullest, our neglect catches up with us and demands payment in full! Cancer, diabetes, arthritis, high blood pressure, and heart failure take their toll. Nuisance illnesses—allergies, colds, indigestion, constipation—meanwhile have their day.

Prevention or Cure?

In a lecture to a medical audience in Doncaster in 1984, Dr. Denis Burkitt said something scary: "I used to labor under the delusion," he admitted, "that doctors and medicine had a profound effect on the health of a community. This I now see as a total fallacy. They have a profound effect on sick people and sick people are very important. But you never reduce the frequency of a disease by improving its treatment. I've had to ask myself . . . Has any disease been reduced significantly because of improved treatment?" With the possible exception of some highly contagious diseases, the answer is, 'No.'

"I spent twenty happy years as a surgeon in Africa," the famed physician soberly recalled. "I enjoyed it all. I helped some people, I hope. I helped to train some African surgeons. But let me be honest. I made no impact whatsoever on the health of the community

I served. If I had spent my twenty years in charge of a team digging wells and latrines I would have done far more for the health of the community.''

So Dr. Burkitt made a change. He reminisces on what he did before and what he has done since:

"I'm not sorry I did what I did, but the point . . . is that it is of little use doing curative medicine unless we are also doing something to prevent disease." He illustrates his point by telling of a cartoon that his daughter drew: Water is running at full force from a tap. The sink is overflowing. Water covers the floor. Some highly dedicated, well-trained, hard-working professionals have arrived in full regalia to take things in hand. Their goal, of course, is to keep the floor dry. Their solution is to mop the floor day and night. They don't even have time for wives and children. It never occurs to them to turn off the faucet. Finally another professional comes by and asks why they didn't turn off the faucet. Here, Dr. Burkitt suggests, we have the modern doctor, dentist or nurse who is becoming more and more oriented to prevention and less and less to cleaning up diseases. He is distressed that he spent thirty years mopping before he found the faucet.

Dr. Burkitt is still regretful that "about 99 percent" of health expenditure in England goes into "floor-mopping" and one percent into turning off taps. He would like to see the day when preventive-medical people will make as good a living as those whose focus is remedial.

The Western Example

Common among the comparisons made by medical missionaries are their stories of the many degenerative diseases common to modern Western culture but practically nonexistent in communities eating traditional foods. Nauru, a small Pacific island only twelve miles around, neatly underscores the differences between the Third World and the West. In 1952 the Island's natives had little degenerative disease such as diabetes and heart trouble. Then large deposits of phosphates were discovered there, and the people, next to the oil-rich Arabs, became the richest in the world.

As they became affluent they adopted Western lifestyles, and before long, 40 percent of the population over age twenty was diabetic. Obesity is now rampant. They now have appendicitis, are expected to develop coronary heart disease, and gallstones also are in prospect.

If you are a philosopher of sorts, you know there are at least two ways to look at living. Some call the first, "altruistic." It is living for the future, for others. The second is today commonly called "narcissistic." It is living only for the here and now, self-centered, indifferent to others. The attitude of the first is "To heaven with me!" and the second beckons you elsewhere. While the results may be delayed, they are as certain as life and death, heaven and hell. And a lack of knowledge is no excuse when the information is available.

The warning, "My people [God's people] are destroyed for lack of knowledge" (Hosea 4:6), is as physical as it is spiritual. Many otherwise godly people are finding out too late that these two cannot be separated without risk.

Modern Pauls

This has special meaning for Christians—and for many Muslims and Jews—for we know that the closer we get to heaven, the more heavenlike our lifestyle will be. Like the apostle Paul, whether he eats or drinks or whatever he does, his first concern is the glory of God (1 Cor. 10:31). His diet will be as near as possible to heaven's diet, his thirst will be quenched by things he will likely find in the New Earth. His daily health plan will be one which builds his body.

We do not offer comfortable, indulgent words, partial truths that go only halfway for fear of colliding with convention. With the help of God and highly qualified internists, health educators, preventive medicine specialists, and nearly fifty years of unusually successful family health, we offer whole truth, logical truth, clinically and scientifically supported truth.

Take care that you do not confuse these truths with conventional living, and turn from them because they are not what most people do. We know that this sounds bold. We also know it works because we have tried it. If you are determined to be logical, read on. If you *happily* adopt the program it suggests, we are certain your life will be much richer and more nearly disease-free. If you are not interested in common sense in health, nor willing to make even *some* of the necessary changes, you will be uncomfortable here. This book will be a pain. Put it down.

Dr. Milton G. Crane, a specialist in hypertension and for many years a teacher in a major medical university, was another physician who, like Dr. Burkitt, became a tap turner. He asked himself a hard question: "What should you do when you know what is causing premature death in over half of your patients and are convinced that you know the cure?" He answered this question by leaving the medical school to enter full-time practice of preventive medicine.

Dr. Crane now administers the widely known lifestyle change program at Weimar Institute* east of Sacramento in Weimar, California. The institute is establishing records in arresting or reversing such degenerative diseases as arthritis, diabetes, heart disease, atherosclerosis, and is helping many in weight control. Although, in his conservative way and for medical reasons, he makes no claims regarding cancer, some of his patients claim remarkable results.

Dr. Crane and his staff of physician specialists, physical therapists, nurses, and other personnel follow all the divine laws described in this book, not diet alone. Yet he singles out animal products and refined foods as the main factors that cause degenerative diseases.

Life Style or Death Style

In assessing what really determines health, these physicians are finding that total *lifestyle* has a greater influence than heredity, environment, and medical science all put together. Recent estimates suggest that the various influences run about like this: Medical 10 percent, Heredity 21 percent, Environment 16 percent, Lifestyle 53 percent. Your lifestyle—or death style—is simply the way you live, and the way you live will determine the kind of health you have. This has been demonstrated by epidemiologic and demographic studies and is often determined by the availability of foods, the social customs of the people, and, most of all, by the degree of "civilization" they have attained. The real meaning of *civilization* is told best by the Bible: about those who would sacrifice present pleasures and those who would not.

---

*Weimar Institute, Box 486, Weimar, CA 95736. [Similar centers include the Black Hills Health and Education Center, Box 1, Hermosa, SD 57744; Hartland Institute, Box 1, Rapidan, VA 22733; Wildwood Sanitarium, Inc. Wildwood, GA 30757, and Uchee Pines Institute, Route 1, Box 273, Seale, AL 36875.] A Weimar patient invented an acrostic for the program NEWSTART, a name that has stuck: N—nutrition, E—exercise, W—water, S—sunshine, T—temperature, A—air, R—rest, and T—trust in God.

But I . . . bring [my body] into subjection.

1 Corinthians 9:27

2

One Man's Reprieve: Trusting and Obeying God

In a book like this which at best is going to make some people unhappy, and at worst will make them angry, it might help to give a first-person, first-hand story of someone who has gone all the way with God in his walk to sound health. And to read Ern Baxter's story is inspiration. So, with the permission of the editors of *New Wine,* let's look at what one man did, one very beloved man of God who describes his "reprieve."

We often run into his picture or hear his name. Not long ago we were guest speakers at the New Covenant Church in Lansing, Michigan where love reigns. We were lodged in their lovely guest house and served our meals by their families, our brothers and sisters. There prominently on the buffet was pictured Ern's happy face.

But Ern is more than a face, and his and Ruth's story is almost as entrancing to us as the raising of Lazarus of Bethany. Only this was nearly 2000 years later than Lazarus, in a day when medical science has little more patience with such stories than did the Pharisees. Ern and Ruth are almost perfect illustrations of the goals of this book. Before you read further, listen to Ern:

As you know, I took on a special assignment the first of the year to serve in a teaching capacity in San Diego. About ten days before

21

my sixty-fifth birthday, I was getting ready to go to my morning teaching assignment and became aware of pressure in my chest. I'd had the first indications of difficulty a few weeks before, but this particular morning it persisted, and Ruth sent for the paramedics. They found my blood pressure alarmingly high and my pulse erratic, so I was taken by ambulance to the hospital where I was thoroughly checked.

Heart Attack Alarm

A cardiologist was called in, and I was put on a telemetry unit— night and day my heart action was monitored. They assured me that I had not had an attack as such, but that all the preliminary symptoms were sufficiently alarming that they wanted me to restrict my activity and to follow a certain regimen. They felt that if the angina (chest pain) continued, it would be advisable for me to submit to an angiogram. If the angiogram was sufficiently severe, I would remain in the hospital and undergo a bypass, a procedure where they take a vein out of your leg and bypass the cloggage.

The angina persisted and I went in for the angiogram, the results of which indicated that the anterior artery in my heart was 70% clogged. The other two arteries—I understand there are three—were in remarkably good shape, but the anterior artery was clogged. However, at that point they didn't feel open-heart surgery was advisable.

After the angiogram, I continued to feel badly and to have angina. I was also under a lot of mental oppression knowing that I had arterial cloggage. You know, when we pass certain milestones in life that have been made famous by tradition, like turning 40 or 50, it can cause stress. I managed forty with a great flourish, and at fifty, my father sent me a fifty dollar bill and said, "Welcome to the fifty club." I handled that great. Sixty didn't seem to be any great problem, either.

But as I approached 65, I came under the influence of the rather universal syndrome of "You're all finished at 65." And to have all this happen ten days before I was 65 only aided and abetted that. So I got caught in that syndrome of hopelessness and futility when you wonder "Should I retire and just sit by and wait?"

Off to Weimar

Interestingly enough, prior to this incident, a brother in northern California, whose wife had had angina as a young woman, had urged me to go to a treatment center called the Weimar Institute because they had helped her tremendously. Ruth and I had agreed to go, and had already made our deposit when I took sick.

So I went to Weimar Institute as kind of a last hope. I had no idea what they were going to do there, only that they had helped my friends. But I wasn't ready for the kind of radical procedure I found.

Weimar Institute is headed by a group of dedicated Christian doctors who are highly trained. They believe that a combination of natural methods can do more to heal a man's problems, promise him longer life and better health, than the more usual route of drugs and surgery. I learned to appreciate these men as highly dedicated, well-qualified men who, in this rather cynical age of ours, demonstrated a degree of dedication above that usually found.

Ruth, incidentally, decided that she would go along and take the treatment as much for my sake as for her own, just so she could help me. And she has been a tremendous help.

When we arrived at the Institute, the first two days were given to orientation. They did blood work and treadmill tests and the whole thing. My blood pressure was elevated, which indicated some problems in that area. I didn't do too well on the treadmill or the cardiogram under stress. Of course, I had been diabetic and was taking insulin by needle, so naturally, when my blood work came back, it indicated that my sugar was elevated, and also that my cholesterol and triglycerides were high. My blood work generally indicated that I had a combination of physical problems.

The next step after the tests was to set up a regimen for me to follow in which my entire day was mapped out for me. The regimen started at 6:30 A.M. with breakfast. There was a medical lecture every morning and devotions. There were some very fine features to this Institute. For example, whenever a physical therapist or hydrotherapist or a medical doctor or a nurse had any occasion to deal with you or do you a service, when they finished, they would have prayer with you, which is rather unique. After you worked out with the physical therapist and he had given you a rubdown, he would say, "Shall we have prayer?"

Right away they put you on a highly personalized nutritional regimen so that everything you eat is monitored by them. I was put on a thousand calories of selected food. They are quite opposed to sugar and all kinds of refined foods and oil. To put it more positively, they major in fruit, vegetables, legumes, and grains.

The Diet

Probably the best explanation is to give my normal daily menu. My breakfast consists of a good portion of hot cereal, toasted specially baked bread and fruit. My lunch consists of vegetables, probably with a bean dish of some kind. My supper consists of fruit and toast (Ruth makes our bread without sugar and without oil, and it's very tasty). There's no eating between meals and no drinking with meals. I can only drink water up to half an hour before I eat, and I don't resume drinking until an hour after. They have a little saying: "At breakfast you eat like a king; at lunch you eat like a queen; and at supper you eat like a pauper." And there's no coffee, of course; no stimulants, no drugs. Between meals, also, we probably drink 7 to 8 glasses of water a day.

With this regimen, within a week or ten days my blood pressure had come down considerably, my weight was starting to come down, and they took me completely off insulin. They took me off all medication, and the only thing now that continues to be somewhat bothersome is a little remaining angina.

Living Again

At the end of the twenty-sixth day, the length of time spent there, blood work was done again. My sugar was down to almost normal. My triglycerides were normalized and my cholesterol was a little below normal. I had taken off ten or twelve pounds and was walking fast four or five miles a day. I was off all my medication, and I was highly motivated. I wanted to live again.

Since leaving there—we've been away about two months—Ruth and I have maintained what they call the therapeutic regimen. We continue pretty much as we did when we were under the treatment at the Institute.

My Ruth

There was one interesting aspect of Ruth's being with me at the institute. Ruth has always taken good care of herself, being a registered nurse, and has maintained a healthy weight level. But we had been pretty heavy meat-eaters and drank a lot of coffee, and one of the alarming things was when they did Ruth's blood work, they found that her triglycerides and cholesterol were higher than mine, and she was bordering on a heart attack. But at the end of our stay at the Institute, her situation had changed considerably.

We're deeply indebted to this program. Although it may be construed as radical or fanatical, anyone who is at all perceptive and informed knows that there is considerable alarm across the nation over the number of heart attacks and strokes and so on. There's a growing concern about the whole nutritional thing.

Sleep

One other side benefit I experienced has to do with sleep. My sleep pattern had been very bad for several years. I generally went to sleep between 12:00 and 1:00 A.M. and woke up at 3:00. Then, if I slept at all the rest of the night, it would be catnapping. Now I go to bed and get six or seven hours sleep which is good for me. I get up in the morning and walk and jog for three miles.

I realize that at sixty-five I can't be twenty-one again, but with this kind of information, I have a desire to use my body—it's kind of a challenge to see how much ground I can regain.

That's pretty much the story of our health pilgrimage. If I may inject a little sermonizing here, my concern would be that young people would do something preventative. It was rather significant to me that all of my fellow patients at the Institute were like myself: they were there because they had either had bypass operations or inoperable heart situations. But isn't it a tragedy that you have to be almost dead before you want to live?

The staff consisted of around ninety people, many of whom were young. They were walking examples of what they were teaching. They were like a bunch of greyhounds. When I looked at those young people who were into this regimen, I thought, "What an opportunity for them in terms of a long healthy life." I wish young people could see this, because I abused my body as a young man. I got away with it for awhile, as most people can, but it finally catches up to you.

During one of the lectures, I mentioned to the doctor that I had heard that a famous professional tennis player—a Wimbledon champion—had had a heart attack at the age of thirty-one. They made it clear to us that being in good physical shape wasn't the total answer. Very simply, the kind of fuel you put into your body determines the internal condition of your body organs. So if I'm going to sermonize a little, I would urge young people to take preventative steps which will promote their physical health and nullify the illnesses that can come as a result of neglecting or mistreating their bodies.

Why Wait?

The sentence that moved us most in Evangelist Ern Baxter's testimony was a single question he asked in the wisdom of retrospection after describing his experience near death: "But isn't it a tragedy that you have to be almost dead before you want to live?"[1] Later, Ern told his full story of healing in an absorbing book, *I Almost Died.*[2] And six years later Walter Martin, a leading Bible scholar, gave a similar testimony after his life-saving experience at the same center—the Weimar Institute at Weimar, California.

This week as we write this, Bill Gothard, the well-known family seminar leader, invited some of us to lunch with him and several of his officials, as he has done for the past several years. This time the conversation centered on the main topic of the day which Bill was presenting to some 1500 area ministers: Health and its relation to the Scriptures, particularly the Old Testament and God's plan for the welfare of His people.

Whether you look at the Old or the New Testaments, whether you are reading Moses or Paul, Bill made it clear that the Bible has much to say about the mental, physical, emotional, and spiritual sides of health. Dorothy started teaching me these things before she became my bride 48 years ago, but it is a new day to have men like Baxter, Martin, and Gothard place *health* in perspective as a privilege and a mandate from God.

Occasionally when friends hear about this book, they chide us with the obvious: "Do you want to take all the joy out of life?"

"What joy?" someone piped up the other night. Turned out it was a woman who has recently undergone a colostomy—so that the residue of her body has to be released from a hole in her side.

So it depends on our values. It is back to our willingness—or refusal—to sacrifice present pleasures for future benefits. Our happy motive is to help you keep pain out of your body and your body out of the grave.

The Savior's Example

This book centers mostly on the physical elements of health. Yet first we must express conviction about the spiritual side. We talk about the grace of Christ, but few of us fully accept in principle or in practice His simple and logical example in daily living—in principle at least, if not precise lifestyle.

We accept His citizenship in heaven.[3] We are in awe that we are sons and daughters of the King, joint-heirs with Christ.[4] We find it hard to wait for the day when we will actually share His throne in the Center of the Universe.[5] We acknowledge that our bodies are temples of the Holy Spirit.[6] And we agree that whether we eat or drink or whatever we do, we should do all to the glory of God![7] *Yet to what extent does our living testimony make these truths our guides in our daily living?*

The Scriptures suggest to us that our God is a fair Judge. He will not hold us responsible for any more than the light we have. Yet when He does express concern, as He does throughout the Bible, you and I dare not treat it as an idle matter. He definitely links the physical and the spiritual: "Beloved," He says, "I wish above all things that thou mayest prosper and be in health, even as thy soul prospereth."[8]

Destroyed for a Lack of Knowledge

If this is all true, and if *we* are true, it may be that we should be more scared of the words of the prophet Hosea who said that

God's "people are destroyed for lack of knowledge." He does not say how they are destroyed, but we might take a hint from physicians who declare that more killing is done in the kitchen and at the dining table than on the highways or in battle.

There is a crucial relationship between sound physical health and the mental, emotional, and spiritual person. They cannot be separated. King Solomon gave us a rare and delightful prescription when he said, "A merry heart doeth good like a medicine." Yet in the same breath he warned that "a broken spirit drieth the bones."[9]

Christ is the great physician. He created the human mind. Even the late dean of American psychiatrists, James T. Fisher, although apparently not a Christian, observed that after searching over the world for material for a handbook on mental health, he found it in the Sermon on the Mount.[10] And if we are looking for examples, it was hardly an accident of fate that the first temptation Satan laid on Christ was on appetite.

Heaven's Lifestyle

It is interesting to us that the best of scientific findings today point more and more to a diet and lifestyle that will be fulfilled in heaven, and as far as possible should be part of our preparations here. To ignore God's way is to adopt the human way. Evangelicals call this "humanism." And whether we do something for ourselves or for God, we have decided in our home that if we do it in our own strength and by our own private standards, we are Pharisees. Theirs was the type of humanism Christ despised above all, and they represented the kinds of characters He will not invite to sit with Him on His throne.

So our prayer these days is to learn of Him in all things and live only to His glory by His grace. For these reasons we study how to eat, how to breathe, how to sleep, how to exercise, and a dozen other areas of health in which we have found that science confirms revelation. We invite you to read this book with the same quest for truth and share the buoyant health and happiness that it has brought to the Baxters and the Martins and us.

3

God's Original Diet

Sometime when you are tinkering with your car or driving along the road, ask yourself which is the most vital—the fuel in the gas tank, the water in the radiator, or the air in the tires. Depending on how far you must go and how much you care about your vehicle, fuel may be first, air second, and water last. Yet you can't go very far if you are out of any of these.

That's the way it is with the body, and with air, water, and food. Here there is also a clear order of priorities. Depending on how long you want to live, air is the most vital, water second, and food third. Yet in terms of *quality* and *quantity,* few of us pay much intelligent attention to any of these. We are influenced more by tradition, peer pressure, advertising, and by habits developed early in life.

Whether or not you are rich or poor or socially prominent in the big city or isolated in the backwoods, usually has little to do with the quality of your nutrition. Malnutrition doesn't necessarily mean that you don't have *enough* to eat. In fact, the richer you are, the more likely you are to have rich food and *poor* nutrition. Your children may be more seriously damaged than you, for the nutritional foundation is built in the years of infancy and childhood, and yours may have been very good. Among many dangers, scientists have found that early severe malnutrition may permanently cripple the immune system—a common concern today.[1]

It is our God-given trust to give our bodies the best available food.[2] If the best available is refined or otherwise of low quality, we can still ask God's blessing on it. But when we can have better nutrition and health, and we choose otherwise, our lifestyle becomes a death style. The blessings we ask at our tables become presumptuous and the surrender we pray for in our daily worship becomes a mockery.

Tuning Your Appetite

Controlling our appetites and health practices is like trying to manage a spoiled child. We are often sneaky, obstinate, inconsistent, rebellious, and hypocritical. And we are so influenced by our peers that we readily sacrifice our principles when we go out. That's the way with a spoiled kid: He will always take advantage of you when company is around. There is probably no "sacrifice" harder for most of us to make than to control the *things* we eat, *how much* we eat, *how often* we eat, *how well* we chew, and our *mealtime state-of-mind*.

Yet the sacrifice is worth making, for we are largely what we eat—often much too large! Any historian, physician or nutritionist can tell that there are two ways to eat, drink, and be merry: for 1) tomorrow we live or 2) tomorrow we die.

You have just bought a new or good used car. You are secretly proud of it, even though you didn't make it. Nevertheless it is your very own, and for a while at least you resolve to give it the best of care. So what do you do to check out its needs? Go to the corner bicycle shop? Talk with the local blacksmith? Hob nob at the junk yard? Never! You get out the owner's manual supplied by your dealer, or you go to the dealer himself. And if you are then not entirely satisfied, you get in touch with the factory representative or with the factory itself. I also did that recently with great satisfaction when I had a fine old Rolleiflex camera that no camera store seemed to understand. I have learned not to tinker around with a fine piece of equipment.

Your body is an infinitely finer piece of equipment than any that man ever made, and deserves the best care you can give it.

Food of most any kind and quality, if not spoiled, may sustain your life temporarily. But to provide life and energy at the highest level, you need a balance of vital substances even more than your car needs gas, oil, grease, water, and air. And since God *made* you, who knows better what will improve the way your human machinery runs?

The Inventor's Prescription

God says simply in Genesis 1:29, "I have given you every herb yielding seed. . . . and every tree, in which is the fruit of a tree yielding seed; to you it shall be for food." Then, after sin came into the world, He also offered "the herb of the field" (Genesis 3:18). In other words, He first provided grains, fruits, nuts—and later vegetables. These are still the Creator's best recipe for healthful living. And He is very serious about this! God permitted appetite to be the first test for man . . . and the first test for Christ.

What do you think when you read how the Savior fed the five thousand from the boy's two fishes and five barley loaves? He could have created an extravagant feast of luxurious foods to gratify their appetites. Yet He chose *the best available food*—the simple fare of the times—to carry out His principle of glorifying His Father by "eating for health and not for drunkenness." But Satan obviously had other ideas than simple, natural foods.

You will notice that no animal products were included in God's ideal diet. We do not understand all the reasons for man's sudden drop in longevity after the Noachian Flood. Yet as he turned from the diet of heaven—when flesh foods were given as an emergency food after vegetation had been destroyed—the lifespan of man dropped from over 900 years to less than 200 in the relatively few generations to Abraham. They eventually dropped to three score and ten—70 years—by New Testament times. We will explore this in more detail in Chapter 8, "Those Vege Nuts."

The Diet Dictators

Even those four simple items which God gave in the beginning—grains, fruits, nuts, and vegetables—have been so depleted by man's meddling that the quality of even a pure vegetarian diet is sometimes questioned. In both Eastern and Western societies we have sleepily allowed the processor—the refiner—to control nutrition and degrade our collective taste buds so that natural foods have little appeal without excess salt, sugar, spices, and other things their Creator hardly intended. But there are signs of an awakening. The U.S. Surgeon General has called for a "public health revolution." He recommends that we eat more whole grains, cereals, fruits, and vegetables. To find specifically how the perversion of these foods affects the body, read on.

Why this sudden change? To get a clear picture, let's take a good look at these items as God made them:

Those Gracious Grains

Probably the most important and abundant food in the diet is the family of seeds of the cereal grasses, used around the world as the staff of life. Rice is the staple for as much as one-third of the world's population and of particular use in Mexico, India, and Asia. Latin America's standby is corn, while millet is most common in northern China. And, of course, we are all well acquainted with wheat. Yet the opportunity for better health and happiness which the use of this nature-fresh, God-given food can bring has been largely destroyed by polishing and bleaching processes and food additives.

These refined grains, though popular in the usual diet and manu-factured largely because they have longer shelf life, are stripped of most of their original vitamins and minerals and dietary fiber. Of more than twenty nutrients which are significantly reduced in the milling process, only thiamine, niacin, riboflavin, and iron are usually added to enrich white flour. The protein quality and fiber are also significantly reduced. Certainly, Isaiah 55:2 applies appropriately to buying white bread, white rice, degerminated corn products, and pasta—spending money on that "which is not bread," and investing labor on that "which does not satisfy" with good health.

When we were living in Japan, Kyoto University's famed rice researcher, Dr. Kondo, told us he believed that most of the vitamins and minerals are lost in the 15 percent of the brown rice kernel milled off to make it white. He ridiculed the rice enrichment process, of which he was principal inventor, as "a sadly inadequate substitute for the real thing." He also reminded us that the Orient was introduced to rice refinement by us—the so-called "civilized" Western World.

Mixing and Preparing Grains

The mixing of grains in cooked cereals or bread produces a higher quality of food value than single grains. That is why we see four, five, six or even seven-grain cereals and breads advertised in health-conscious stores. Use at least two or three kinds of whole grains each day in your diet. They provide what might be called a "synergistic" effect: They bring to you more nutrition when mixed than the sum of them when eaten separately.

You will also need to note the proper preparation of cereals. This is especially true for infants under one year of age. Grains, in contrast to fruits and most vegetables (excepting dry beans), need long, slow cooking. In the case of harder grains, several hours is best. See the chart on whole grain cookery.

The loss of needed vitamins, minerals, and even protein from refined grains is a serious enough loss. Yet the lack of fiber in refined grains is probably an even more devastating problem. Since refined foods other than grains also have had fiber removed and because the different types of fiber have different functions, fiber will be discussed in more detail under Elimination in Chapter 11.

Healing Fruit

Certainly fruit will be among the main treats of heaven, picked fresh from the Tree of Life with its twelve fruits, and possibly many more. How does our appetite react when we ask, What is more delicious than a fresh apple or orange or apricot or pear or papaya or mango or pineapple or grape picked directly from the tree or vine or plant? Fruits seldom disagree with our stomachs, unless we have abused them.

Summer brings its many kinds of berries, and fall with its apples and peaches and pears is the largest fruit production time, depending on which side of the equator you live. Then there are the citrus fruits, bananas, avocados, and others which appear at random times, depending on the location and climate and nature of the fruit. But, are you aware that most of us can now have a variety of fresh fruit all the year round?

There are many advantages to the use of simple fresh fruits. They cleanse the body internally and avoid several health-destroying practices (such as refined sugar, refined fats, cholesterol, salt, and high calories). They seldom have to be cooked—saving gas, electricity, and a lot of work. And they may easily be frozen or canned with minimum nutritional loss.

When we were missionaries in Japan, it was Dorothy's happy task each night to set a big bowl of fresh fruit in the middle of the table. She saw to it that each of us had a fruit knife to prepare his own fruit. It was easier for her and fun for us all. Besides, it was delicious, and healthful—and disease-free! The simple idea of all doing the same thing at the same time—cutting and coring— made those suppers special times. And there were few, if any,

WHOLE GRAIN COOKERY

Amount of Grain	Water	Salt	Boil 1–2 Minutes Then Lower Heat. Cover Tightly. Do not Remove Lid While Cooking	Yield
½ c. hulled barley	2 c.	¼ t.	45 min.	2¼ c.
½ c. buckwheat groats	1 c.	¼ t.	15 min.	2½ c.
1 c. millet	4 c.	½ t.	30–35 min.	4 c.
1 c. oat groats*	3 c.	¾ t.	1 hour	2½ c.
1 c. brown rice	2 c.	½ t.	40–45 min. Let stand 10 min.	2½ c.
½ c. whole rye*	2½ c.	¼ t.	6 hours	2¼ c.
½ c. triticale**	1½ c.	¼ t.	1 hour & 30 min.	1⅔ c.
1 c. red cereal wheat*	4 c.	½ t.	6–8 hours	2½ c.
1 c. cornmeal	4 c.	¼ t.	20–25 min.	3½ c.
1 c. rolled oats	2 c.		20–25 min.	1¾ c.
1 c. whole wheat berries*	3 c.	1 t.	2 hours	2⅔ c.

** *Triticale* is a new grain crossed between wheat and rye with higher protein than either.
* Soak dry grain overnight. (To shorten cooking and soaking time, bring to a rolling boil, cover. Turn off heat and let stand one hour.)
Two important secrets in cooking cereals with delicious flavor are:
  1. Allow enough water to swell and soften all the starch.
  2. Cook them long enough. Slow, thorough cooking softens the cellulose more and develops the flavor of the starch.
  3. Toasting (dextrinizing) in dry skillet, stirring constantly, or in the oven seems to bring out the flavor and hasten cooking time.
Steaming in a double boiler, rice cooker, crock pot, etc., takes almost double cooking time. A little more water can be added. Grains vary. Buckwheat absorbs a double amount of water when steamed. Steaming is an excellent way to reheat cooked cereals. Steaming can also be done in the oven.

Source: Weimar Institute, P.O. Box 486, Weimar, CA 95736

dishes to do! Occasionally we added zwiebach—made by drying rough whole-grain bread in the oven. Chewed thoroughly, it becomes a natural sweet and quickly digests.

Nutritious Nuts

God made these unique foods for us to balance our diets. But you will notice that they were often put in a hard shell, so they are a little difficult to prepare. Do you remember the old-fashioned nut bowl with the nutcracker in it? You were not likely to overeat when you had to crack all you ate yourself. Could it be that because of their high concentration of protein and fat, God packaged nuts so that they would be used in moderation? See Protein in Chapter 6.

Almonds and walnuts may be among our most commonly used and perhaps most valuable nuts. Cashews, brazil nuts, pecans, macadamia nuts, and especially coconuts should be used a little more sparingly, because of their high-fat content. This is also true of peanuts, which are legumes (like beans and peas) and really aren't nuts at all. While peanut butter is a favorite of many, it should be used sparingly. If you have a tendency to use a good deal of peanut butter, try diluting it by emulsifying it (mixing it with water) and spreading it thinly. Yet remember that when so emulsified, it does not keep well, so you may want to prepare only a little at a time.

Valuable Vegetables

These foods have long been accepted as valuable, but they are coming into increasing demand as science has become more informed about nutrition. Carotene and Vitamin A, for example, which are plentiful in red, green, and yellow vegetables, have recently been found to repress cancer even in smokers and drinkers. Regina G. Ziegler presented studies of 1,000 people at a 1985 American Cancer Society forum in Daytona Beach, Florida.[3]

The British medical journal, *Lancet,* told of a similar study done over a period of 19 years in the Chicago area. And Dr. Takeshi Hirayama of Japan reported in a radio interview results of a study covering 16 years of observation of 265,118 people (*Fresh Report on Family Hour,* Summer 1985). Ziegler added that diet changes, of course, cannot eliminate the risks of using tobacco and alcohol. Dr. Hirayama further noted that the group which abstained from meat, as well as tobacco and alcohol, had the lowest rate of cancer.

The *Lancet* also warned against the use of Vitamin A supplements, because too much can cause liver damage. Red, green or yellow fruits and vegetables do not create such hazards. They include carrots, beets, tomatoes, dark salad greens, yellow squash, sweet potatoes or yams, broccoli, peaches, persimmons, grapes, and apples.

Unfortunately, many people turn from vegetables even though they know they are healthful. Yet we do not always blame them. Part of the problem may lie in the method used in caring for and cooking them. This has much to do with maintaining the vitamins, minerals, and delicious flavor which are available in these valuable foods.

First, bad treatment of vegetables consists of peeling them, letting them sit around at room temperature after being picked, soaking them in water, and even boiling them long and hard in lots of water and then pouring off the water into the drain.

Cooking Cautions

Now what's so bad about this kind of treatment?

Peeling causes considerable loss of minerals which are concentrated just under the skin. Peeling, for example, allows oxygen to destroy Vitamin C, and other valuable nutrients are totally peeled away. Loss in peeling a potato may range from 12 to 35 percent of the Vitamin C. The skin of carrots is rich in thiamin, niacin, and riboflavin.[4] Only when the skin is tough, bitter or impossible to clean thoroughly, should you peel vegetables. Otherwise, just scrub them well with a vegetable brush.

Discarding the outer leaves of vegetables also deprives you of higher concentrations of vitamins and minerals than are found in inner, though more tender, leaves. In the green outer leaves of cabbage, for example, are approximately 2–3 times as much iron, almost twice as much vitamin C and 21 times more vitamin A as in the bleached inner ones. Yet your vegetable market usually strips off most of the best part, often saving it to make healthy hogs, and when you remove the remaining outer leaves you may remove much of the remainder. Lettuce and other green vegetables are much the same.[5]

The lesson is clear both in choosing and preparing leafy vegetables! If you find it really necessary to cut away some of these valuable trimmings, try simmering them into a broth to be used for gravy or soup. Ask your vegetable man if he can let you have some unstripped heads.

Soaking, either while waiting to be washed, or in a pan waiting to be cooked or overcooking, causes the greatest loss in nutrients. Even four minutes of hard boiling causes losses of 20–45 percent of total minerals, 75 percent of natural sugars, and still greater losses of some vitamins. Soaking or delayed washing in cold water causes some loss in water-soluble nutrients and natural flavors. If vegetables were people, they would cry "Criminal!" at cooks who treat them this way. There are good ways to treat these friends to insure that you keep as much as possible of the nutrition God put into them:

Natural and Fresh

Look always for freshness. You can't beat your own garden or that of a friend, relative or neighbor where you can bring your produce from your field to your kitchen in the shortest possible time. Otherwise, learn what days new produce comes in at your market. Don't overbuy so that vegetables will lose nutrients from aging. Generally leave them not more than three to five days in your refrigerator. Don't keep them in the car, on the sink, or even in water until you "get around" to washing them. Get them into the refrigerator where it's dark, cold, and humid. Plastic bags or containers even within your vegetable bin help maintain the best humidity to keep them from wilting. Fresh tomatoes are probably the only vegetables which do not need that humidity.

We have no burden to encourage a diet—adopted by many—of eating only what you can eat raw. Yet you will do well to serve some raw vegetables at your vegetable meals and fresh fruits at your other meals. You need a variety of nutrients, and it is true that some foods are more easily digested when cooked, such as beans, beets, potatoes, and winter squash.

People who have not learned to enjoy cooked vegetables will often eat most of them best when raw. Dorothy often brings me a small plate of "rabbit food," as I call it, while she is finishing the preparation of our main meal. Happily I munch on raw carrots, celery, broccoli, a wedge of cabbage or lettuce, kale or whatever she has on hand. Because I am hungry before mealtime, I look forward to this appetizer course, relish these vegetables more, and I have lots of time to chew and chew.

Except for therapeutic purposes when your health has been seriously damaged by illness, accident or mistreatment, vegetable juices are not a cure-all either. In general, eat your food in as natural a form as possible and prepared in the best way you can to get all available nutrients—just enough "fixing" to reveal their best qualities.

Keeping It Simple

Many people these days are learning that to maintain food value, color, and flavor, the Chinese method of stir-frying where the vegetables are cooked quickly until just tender but crispy, is the best. The Chinese start with oil, but you can achieve the same effect without oil, and even without a Chinese *wok,* but with just a little water on the bottom of the pan.

Dorothy often cooks vegetables this way, usually in a frying pan since we never use it to "fry" any more—especially in one that is teflon or Silverstone. She usually does not use any more water than is on the vegetables when they are washed, although she occasionally adds a tablespoon or two if it is necessary. If she turns the heat down soon after the pan is hot and she watches and stirs frequently, she finds that she needs little or no water with most quick-cooking vegetables.

Shredded cabbage, greens, zucchini, and other summer squashes are delicious this way. Since I like onions in almost everything, she often cuts or slices an onion with these. Then she seasons them with garlic and perhaps a pinch or two of herbs—and I hardly miss the salt.

With longer-cooking vegetables, she almost always steams them with a tight-fitting lid to avoid oxidation from the air and saves the water for soup, gravy or to cook legumes. Otherwise she microwaves them without any water at all. While there is no perfect cooking method, she sometimes uses the pressure cooker with its rack as a steamer but generally reserves pressure cooking only for emergencies because the high temperature it requires may destroy vitamins. And we don't want to destroy our friends!

4

Carbohydrates—The Fuel in Your Tank

Between us, Dorothy and I have a century of experience in teaching. This has taught us that changing basic habits comes usually in three or four ways: 1) a life-threatening emergency, 2) emulation of a hero, 3) love and respect such as you will find in a good marriage, and 4) thinking to principle and living by it. How are *you* motivated? Why do you do what you do? Are you in control of your lifestyle? Or does it control you?

Knowing the whys and hows of diet—the content and use of foods and how and why they affect you—puts you in better control of both your health and happiness. You don't have to get technical about it, but just know what is right, and its effect on your body. The whys are the principles, the *basic reasons why,* and they give you clear, thoughtful direction. In other words, the principles—*knowing why we do what we do*—provide incentives. Here are some interesting facts which may help you do this:

Those Sugars

Natural *carbohydrates* come in two forms: 1) simple (sugars) and 2) complex (starches). They include fiber, as do all natural foods. They are needed for energy, body warmth, cleansing the

38

body by laxative action and removing toxic materials, and for nerve and brain function. They are found in every plant food, especially in fruits and cereals. You should normally obtain about 70 to 80 percent of your calories from these in their natural form.

When refined, however, *sugar* becomes a spoiler. It is not your friend. It sneaks many health problems into you, such as food sensitivities, obesity, dental decay, hypoglycemia, diabetes, heart disease, and lowered resistance to infection. Sugar is so sneaky, in fact, so well hidden in almost all prepared foods, that few of us realize it is there. Our use of sugar has skyrocketed in the last 200 years in the United States.

Honey

Even *honey* is not as friendly as many think. It should not be used *freely* as a substitute for refined sugar, for it is also "refined" in its own way—*by the bees for bees*. It is nearly twice as sweet as sugar, and so high in energy that some nutritionists call it "jet fuel"—for bees.

Many health enthusiasts have absorbed or preached the gospel that honey is superior to sugar. And we certainly don't want to be kill-joys. Yet we feel compelled to report that certain well-documented facts have been established to question honey's widely touted superiority: Although honey does have minute amounts of some essential minerals such as potassium, calcium, and phosphorus, they are not significant in your diet. Honey and sugar have about the same number of calories. On the one hand fructose in honey is better for diabetics than the sucrose in sugar; yet, on the other hand, raw (unprocessed) honey may contain botulism spores in quantities sufficient to cause food poisoning in babies less than a year old. If it is processed, many of the trace minerals are essentially lost.[1]

After the above information was printed in the Tufts *Diet and Nutrition Letter*, some readers objected strongly, insisting that honey contains important nutrients. They obviously didn't want their fantasy balloon to burst. Yet the amounts of trace elements are so small that they have little value in nutrition. One tablespoon of honey produces less than one percent of the U.S. Recommended Daily Allowance of a single nutrient.

Fruit Juices

Even *unsweetened fruit juice* is refined. One glass of apple juice, for example, is extracted from at least three to five apples. Its sugars go more directly into the bloodstream than do those of the fresh fruit itself, because its cellulose packaging has been removed. This raises the blood-sugar level rapidly, especially if taken between meals. (See Chapter 14 "The 5 R's—Part II" for more on snacking.) *Dried fruit* does have much to commend it, yet not as a between-meal snack. It is so highly concentrated that it should also be used in limited amounts, unless it is used in the meal as a principal source of calories—as a main dish.

Sugar and Infections

But you have a right to ask how and why sugar is so unfriendly. And we reply that one of the main functions of our white blood cells is to fight off *infection*. They are the body's soldiers. One white blood cell normally can destroy fourteen harmful bacteria in half an hour. After you eat one cup of ice cream—usually containing six teaspoons of sugar—your white blood cells each can destroy only four to ten bacteria. If you eat a banana split with its usual twenty-five teaspoons of sugar, your white blood cells can each eliminate only one germ.

So if you wonder why respiratory infections are rampant, and *tooth decay* is common, and why you or your friends are so often vulnerable to colds and other diseases, make an honest check, and close the door on sugar-dosed foods. Don't be like King Belshazzar's men who left Babylon's river gates open and simplified Cyrus' problem of conquering the city. Dare instead to be a Daniel, who with his friends set the stage for world history by first conquering his appetites.

Carbohydrates and Your Teeth

Tooth decay affects more than 95 percent of the American people, yet it is preventable. Chemically speaking, teeth are stable enough to last a lifetime and sometimes do, especially in simple societies where food is eaten mostly in its natural form. Proper cleaning of your teeth obviously does make a difference, but that is not enough.

Anything that affects your nutritional balance influences the health of your teeth.

For many reasons refined sugar is the main villain in tooth decay. For example, it lacks phosphorus, where in its natural form in sugar cane you will find this important mineral. Also, sugar in whole fruit or other whole foods is usually combined with phosphorus. A lack of this mineral directly contributes to tooth decay.[2]

It has also long been known that the *frequency* of eating sugared foods and drinks is very significant in the development of cavities in teeth.[3] It seems that the destructive bacterium, *Streptococcus mutans,* lodges in the plaque deposits which accumulate on your teeth. In the presence of sugar it produces lactic acid which eats into your teeth, drilling those unwanted holes. Generally speaking, your susceptibility to dental caries is in direct proportion to the amount of this acid in your normally alkaline saliva. On the other hand, healthy, acid-free saliva washes the teeth externally to maintain them in excellent condition. Any food eaten between meals, especially those which stick to the teeth, including dried fruit, promotes tooth decay.

That Ominous Snacking

When rats are given one high-sugar meal, their output of parotid hormone is decreased eightfold. Drs. Steinman and Leonora further conclude that between-meal snacking is one of the worst, and possibly the worst, of all inducers of tooth decay. Even one between-meal snack can induce a twenty to thirty-minute acid attack on the precious enamel of your teeth.[4] Their conclusions are strongly supported by a Stockholm, Sweden study of 400 patients over a five-year period.[5] The sweeter, the stickier, and the oftener sweets are eaten, along with a poor quality of basic diet, the more damage the sugar will cause.

Keeping It Simple

Tooth decay dropped dramatically during World War II as shown by dental records of Denmark, Finland, and Norway, during the years 1938 to 1945. With a 50 percent drop in sugar consumption—from 80 to 40 pounds per capita in some areas—came a decline from 90 percent incidence of cavities in children before the War, to 25 percent at War's end. Also whole grain cereals often replaced refined cereals for economy's sake.[6] Similar studies were done in the U.S., Japan, and other areas with equivalent results.[7]

Though the people returned to their pre-war diet after the war, the tooth decay in seven-year-old Norwegian children continued to decline for seven more years until in 1952 only 10 percent of the seven-year-olds had tooth decay. Dr. R. F. Sognnaes and other researchers concluded that the good diet not only reduced cavities in the children already born, but provided sound teeth to children whose mothers were "limited" to this better diet during war-time pregnancy. He also experimented with animals with similar results.[8]

When your diet contains a high proportion of refined sugar of any kind, your blood sugar rises in only a few minutes, because refined sugar is absorbed promptly. This in turn brings on a surge of insulin to deal with the sugar. The blood sugar then drops to a lower level than before the food was eaten, whetting the appetite for more food. You can easily bring on a roller-coaster blood sugar level with the common diet of coffee and sugar or sweet roll before rushing to the office, another coffee or coke with doughnut or sweet roll at midmorning, a coke for lunch, a candy bar midafternoon, a heavy dinner, and a snack before bedtime. This often produces *hypoglycemia*, a condition in which your blood sugar falls so low that you feel weak, headachy, and "down" in your thinking.

Those Naturally Packaged Sweets

Yet this does not happen so easily with natural sweets unless you overdo or eat between meals. God wrapped His sweets in fiber and other components so that the sugar is absorbed more slowly and holds the blood level steady for a longer time. High sugar intake is also associated with adult-onset *diabetes* which makes up 80 percent of diabetic patients. The other 20 percent are childhood-onset, which researchers do not yet well understand.

Fortunately there is hope for these victims. Adult-onset diabetes can usually be reversed by a lifestyle change. Among other things, they must first *eliminate* refined sugar and visible fats. Then it is important to add whole grains because of the crucially important fiber they contain and to avoid the loss through the refining process of 60 to 70 percent of their natural trace elements such as chromium, zinc, manganese, copper, and vanadium. These very items, so important in maintaining normal blood sugar balance, are milled out in the refining process.[9]

Heart Disease and Obesity

Researchers have recently found that substantial sugar intake—especially with cholesterol and saturated fat—increases the serum triglyceride levels of the blood, a condition which may be as conducive to heart disease as abnormally high cholesterol. Few realize that sugar is also rapidly converted in the liver to fat (triglycerides) which is still another factor in heart disease and *obesity*.

Sugar in its unnatural, refined state performs unnatural acts. Like any perversion—sexual or dietary—it is never truly creative. Instead it offers empty calories because important vitamins and minerals are gone, including vitamin B_1, riboflavin, and niacin. Yet to be metabolized and to be properly absorbed into the body, it must have these minerals. So sugar robs the body of these nutrients which were put there by other foods. When this happens, the body is weakened, often with serious results, and the deficiencies have an effect on the emotions, behavior, morals, and logically and ultimately, mental health.

Sweets and Behavior

This linkage between sugar and crime shouldn't be surprising, for refined sugar is itself a robber, a criminal. Alexander Schauss, Director of the Institute of Biosocial Research in Tacoma, Washington, says that while all criminals aren't sugar freaks, and all sugar freaks don't have antisocial or criminal tendencies, nearly half the criminals in the country eat their way into prison. In certain individuals the metabolic imbalance caused by abnormal consumption of refined sugar tends to induce erratic behavior. Some eat as much as 465 pounds a year, nearly four times the already high American average.

Strange as it may seem, the fewer the sweets, the sweeter the disposition. Proverbs 23:1 and 3 reminds us that "When thou sittest to eat with a ruler, consider diligently what is before thee. . . . Be not desirous of his dainties: for they are deceitful meat." Also David's prayer in Psalm 141:3, 4 is appropriate: "Set a watch, O

Lord, before my mouth; keep the door of my lips . . . : and let me not eat of their dainties.''

Stoking Your Body Stove

Sugar is also habit-forming and develops unnatural cravings as well as destroying your taste or appetite for nutritious foods. This is one sound rationale for serving dessert at the *end* of the meal after the stomach is well filled, and helps at least a bit in avoiding overweight. Eventually you will be ''all stopped up,'' for along with other low residue foods, sugar also promotes constipation.

Here are some approximate amounts of sugar in the average ''harmless'' drink or dessert:

Can of soft drink	12 oz.	7–10 tsp.
Lemonade	8 oz.	7 tsp.
Cocoa	8 oz.	4 tsp.
Applesauce, sweetened	1 cup	9 tsp.
Jell-o	½ cup	5 tsp.
Pie	average piece	5–12 tsp.
Glazed doughnut	one	7 tsp.
Cake	4 oz. piece	10 tsp.
Ice cream	½ cup	5 tsp.
Hard candy	1 oz.	7 tsp.
Canned peaches, sweetened	2 halves	3 tsp.
Wheaties or Total	1 oz.	1 tsp.
Cocoa Krispies	1 oz.	3 tsp.

Whatever your motivation for eating, at least stoke your body's furnace with as good judgment as you would your fine wood stove. You would never burn materials that would permanently tar or clog your chimney, nor fuel that would burn so hot that it would crack your stove. Nor would you be careless about the gasoline you put in your tank—unless you couldn't care less about your car. Yet your chimney, stove, and car can be replaced; your body is all you have. So . . . be careful about the fuel you put in your tank!

5

Fat—That Dual Personality—and His Bride Cholesterol

A man who had undergone heart by-pass surgery several years previously told Dorothy his dramatic story of recovery when she was at Weimar. After he left the hospital, the doctors had cautioned him briefly about not eating too many eggs and getting some exercise, but somehow it wasn't enough. In about five or six years, he was back to the same doctors with the same seriously clogged blood vessels. They then told him that he would not be able to stand another surgery and, for all practical purposes, just to go home and enjoy life for the few months he might have left.

Someone suggested he go to a chelation therapist to have his blood vessels cleaned out by intravenous medicines. He promptly sought out a doctor who practiced this therapy. But to the physician's credit, he told him that chelation would not do him any good.— What he needed was *permanent* chelation and the best place to go was Weimar Institute. At the time Dorothy talked with him it was almost two years since he had gone through the lifestyle change at Weimar. He was not only enthusiastic, but even jubilant, about how good he felt and how he loved that place. He and his wife have a motor home, are staying on the program, and have dedicated their lives to spreading the gospel of health. They have no particular religion or creed otherwise, but believe in the lifestyle because it works.

Our best information is that tablets taken by mouth, medicines induced into the blood vessels or any other method which is not consistent with God's natural laws are seldom, if ever, permanent cures or even effective whether used for preventive or remedial purposes. Recently the Food and Drug Administration has ordered four manufacturers to remove such heart pills from the market and warned consumers not to take them. On the other hand, correct habits of eating and living have been shown to be safe, successful, and acceptable both in maintaining health and in reversing health problems.

Those Hidden Fats

One of the worst enemies of our blood carriers is the overuse of fat. We have the choice of continuing in this dietary error (about which all health educators are concerned and trying to find remedies like chelation) or to use fat in the right way and never have to deal with its misuse.

Fatty acids are of three types and are found in all fats we eat. These fatty acids combine with glycerols to form triglycerides or fat. The classifications are: (1) *saturates,* more plentiful in animal products than in plant foods (2) *monounsaturates,* primarily oleic and extremely important to your health and; (3) *polyunsaturates.* The latter two are of both animal and vegetable origin and mostly liquid at room temperature, except for those which have been hydrogenated. Fats supply energy and help keep skin smooth and healthy by supplying these fatty acids. They are major components of every cell membrane, and are raw material for four families of very important body chemicals. And they also carry vitamins A, D, E, and K. Fat is found in natural form in all foods such as fruits, grains, nuts, and vegetables. You will even find some in such unlikely foods as lettuce or grapefruit.

From these plant foods, many medical and nutritional specialists now are convinced, it is possible to get all the fat you normally need without any animal fat or added vegetable fat at all. We do not suggest that you suddenly dump all your cooking oils, but we do recommend you study the possibility that the more closely you linger with foods in their natural forms, the more likely you will have buoyant health.

When Less Is Better

To *prevent* disease, the *ideal* proportion for a young, healthy person should be not more than 15 percent to 35 percent of your daily calory intake in fats, and then *only with fat in its natural form*. Yet if you have a family history of heart disease, or if you or your family have weight or other health problems such as atherosclerosis, diabetes or high blood pressure (hypertension), a prevention oriented physician may limit your calories of fat to no more than 10 or 15 percent. This means that even the use of such high-fat natural foods as avocadoes, nuts, olives, and soy beans may be sharply limited or not be used at all for several months or until you are well on the way to recovery.

In any case, be sure to continue periodic blood tests and take seriously any other symptoms which suggest a stricter regimen. We add these cautions in the belief that true temperance is abstinence of all harmful things and careful use of all that are natural and good.

The average person in the Western world consumes more than three times the proportion of his energy from fat than does one who lives in the several populations of the Third World. In Aboriginal societies, for example, where the diet includes only 10 to 20 percent of the total calories in fat, it is also low in animal products, and where salt is less than 5 grams a day, cholesterol averages 150 (ranging from 110 to 180). Though afflicted with some infections, aborigines have little *coronary heart disease* and very little diabetes or high blood pressure.

Lessons from Japan

The influence of heredity has been largely ruled out in a study of the Japanese lifestyle as the major factor in heart disease. Japanese natives whose diet consists of about 10 percent fat showed an average serum cholesterol of 150. Yet Japanese in Hawaii with 25 percent fat in their diets, showed cholesterol averages of 220 and had four times the relative death rate from coronary heart disease as those in Japan. Worse still, Los Angeles Japanese with a dietary fat content of 40 percent and cholesterol average of 250 had nine times the relative death rate of those in Japan.[1]

Reading Labels

Become an avid "label reader" and estimate about how much fat—and other elements—you are eating, by checking the labels on the prepared foods you buy. One *gram* of fat is equal to *nine* calories. So you should multiply the *grams* of fat per serving times *9* to find the *calories* of fat per serving. Calories of fat per serving divided by total calories in one serving equals the percentage of fat. For example, if the label says that one serving is 135 calories and that there are 5 grams of fat, you know that 45 calories of that serving—or 33 percent—are fat.

Don't be fooled by lowfat dairy products which say "2% milkfat, 98% fat free." These are indeed better for you than whole-milk products, but look what you get if you check the label and figure it out. One lowfat cottage cheese label we checked with the above advertisement on the cover, listed the contents thus: A ½ cup serving equals 100 calories with two grams of fat. That means that 18 calories of the 100, or 18 percent of the ½ cup of cottage cheese is fat as measured in calories.

Similarly, when you want to know the percentage of calories from protein or carbohydrate in a particular food, multiply the number of grams in a serving by *4* to find the number of calories

PERCENT of CALORIES AS FAT IN FOOD

Food	%	Food	%
Milk, whole	52	Butter	97
Ice cream	55	Margarine	99
Eggs	64	Shortening	100
Cheddar Cheese	72	Most cereal grains	5
Cream Cheese	90	Oats	10–15
Beef, average	70	Corn	10
Hamburger	74	Fruits (most)	1
Pork, lean	70	Vegetables	1–5
Milk chocolate	60	Legumes (except soy)	5
Potato chips	61	Nuts	60–90

Caculated from U.S.D.A. "Composition of Foods," Agriculture Handbook No. 8.

Source: Weimar Institute, P.O. Box 486, Weimar, CA 95736

and then determine your percentage by dividing that number by the total number of calories per serving. For example, on one cereal box we read "110 calories per 1 oz. serving." Protein is 4 grams. Multiply this number—4—by four, which gives you 16, meaning 16 calories out of the 110 are protein, or 14.5 percent.

Take another example: On a package of nonfat powdered milk we find that a cup of reconstituted liquid milk contains 80 calories. Eight grams are protein, and when multiplied by four, you have 32 calories of protein or 40 percent (32 divided by 80). And in that case nonfat does indeed mean no calories in fat.

The Pretender

Fat pretends to be your friend, and when kept in its place, it does some very good things for you. But it wants most all of your attention, and will turn your other friends off if you aren't careful. We find so much of it, especially in animal products, that it makes up at least 45 to 50 percent of the calories in whole milk, 64 percent in eggs, 74 percent in hamburger, 90 percent in cream cheese, and about 98 percent in butter or margarine. This may help you better understand how easily you can raise your average fat intake to the dangerous levels in the typical American diet where the average proportion of calories of fat in your food is 40 percent or more.

Watching Limits

The American Heart Association suggests a limit of 30 percent, with no more than one-third of this in saturated (animal) fat, but that is still a poor compromise with the ideal. Remember that these saturates are *empty calories* without minerals, vitamins, and fiber. And fat is far more devious than most of us imagine.

Furthermore, it's impossible to discuss fat without involving *cholesterol* because the percentage of saturated or animal fat and polyunsaturated or free fat in the diet is generally recognized as the lead villain in the drama of heart disease, the number one killer in the United States. In 1984 the Federal Government report of the broadest and most expensive research project in medical history confirmed that the cholesterol level in our bloodstream is directly affected by the richness of our diet. Heart disease was found to be specifically related to the amount of cholesterol in the blood and that "for every 1 percent reduction in total cholesterol level, there is a 2.4 percent reduction of heart-disease risk."[2]

What about Cholesterol?

Cholesterol is not all bad. It contributes to insulation around the nerve fibers as, for example in the myelin or covering of nerve tissue in the brain. Sunshine performs the miracle of irradiating the cholesterol in our skin into Vitamin D. One of the main roles of bile salts—a derivative of cholesterol—is to process fat. The liver manufactures cholesterol in response to dietary fat and converts about 70 percent of it into bile salts. Some of the bile is concentrated in the gall bladder and released at mealtime to emulsify the fat in our intestines. Since every cell in our bodies makes cholesterol, it is not necessary to add more from the food we eat (see how snacking interferes with this process in Chapter 14, The Five R's, Part II).

LDL and Dangerous Cholesterol

First, there is an ingredient in the little balls of food fat in the blood, called *low-density lipoprotein* (LDL). An excess of LDL can deliver an excess of fat and cholesterol to the cells. The higher the level of LDL, the higher the risk of atherosclerosis. It is increased by such foods as eggs, cheese—or, for that matter, any vegetable

EFFECT OF EMPTY CALORIES ON A MEAL

Food	Calories	Calories
Lettuce & Tomato Salad	20 + Mayonnaise (80)	100
Bread	60 + Butter (60)	120
Peas	100 + Butter (60)	160
Entree	150 + Gravy (100)	250
Baked Potato	100 + Butter (60)	160
Skimmed Milk	80 Whole Milk	160
Baked Apple	90 Apple Pie ⅙	350
	600	1,300

Source: Weimar Institute, P.O. Box 486, Weimar, CA 95736

APPROXIMATE AMOUNTS OF CHOLESTEROL IN FOODS

Food		Cholesterol (mg)
Meat: Beef, lamb, pork, veal, 3 oz, 1 pc 4x2x½" retail cuts, cooked, without bone		30
Liver, 3 oz		370
Kidneys, 3 oz		675
Poultry:		
Chicken, breast, meat & skin, 3 oz, ½ breast		74
" , " , without skin from a 3 lb chicken		63
" , 1 drumstick, meat & skin, 2 oz		47
" , " , without skin from a 3 lb chicken		39
Turkey, light, without skin, 3 oz, 2 pcs 4x2x½"		65
" , dark, without skin		86
Fish & Seafood:		
Clams	1 cup, 19 large	114
Crab	1 cup, canned, packed	161
Lobster	1 cup, cut in ½" cubes	123
Oysters	1 cup, 19–31 medium	120
Shrimp	1 cup, 22 large or 76 small	192
Halibut, broiled, 3 oz		50
Salmon, broiled, 3 oz		35
Sardines, drained solids, 3¼ oz net wt		129
Dairy Products:		
Butter, regular	½ oz, 1 Tbsp	35
Buttermilk, cultured, nonfat	8 oz, 1 cup	5
Cheeses		
Cheddar, milk or sharp	1 oz, 1" cube	28
Ricotta (part skim)	1 oz, 1" cube	9
Cottage, creamed (4% fat)	8 oz, 1 cup packed	48
" , uncreamed	8 oz, 1 cup packed	13
Cream cheese	½ oz, 1 Tbsp	16
Cream		
Half and half	½ oz, 1 Tbsp	6
Light coffee or table	½ oz, 1 Tbsp	10
Sour cream	½ oz, 1 Tbsp	8
Whipped topping	1.2 oz, ¼ cup (pressurized)	13
Heavy whipping	½ oz, 1 Tbsp (unwhipped)	20
Ice Cream, regular	2½ oz, ½ cup	20
Ice Milk, hardened	2½ oz, ½ cup	13
Milk		
Whole	8 oz, 1 cup	34
Low fat (2% fat)	8 oz, 1 cup	22
Nonfat	8 oz, 1 cup	5
Yogurt, from fluid & dry nonfat milk	8 oz, 1 cup	17
Eggs:		
Whole	1 large	252
Yolk	1 large	252
Deserts:		
Cakes		
Sponge	2¼ oz, 1/12 of 10" diam. cake	162
Yellow, chocolate frosting	2½ oz, 1/16 of 9" diam. cake	36
Angel food	2 oz, 1/12 of 10" diam. cake	0
Cream puffs with custard	4½–5 oz, 3.5" diam.	188
Custard, baked	8 oz, 1 cup	278
Pies, baked (vegetable-oil crust)		
Custard	⅛ of 9" diam. pie	120
Fruit	1 piece	0
Lemon meringue	⅛ of 9" diam. pie	98
Pumpkin	⅛ of 9" diam. pie	70
Puddings, cooked		
Chocolate or vanilla	8 oz, 1 cup	32
Salad Dressings:		
Mayonnaise, commercial	½ oz, 1 Tbsp	10
Fruit:	any amount	0
Nuts:	any amount	0
Grains:	any amount	0
Vegetables:	any amount	0
Legumes: (peas, beans)	any amount	0

Developed from U.S. Department of Agriculture and other bulletins.

or animal fats. It is commonly known that preparing foods with oils and greases tends to build an abnormally high cholesterol level.

This also explains the dangers of one of my favorite foods, processed cheese—American, Swiss, Jack, and so on. Cheese, an animal product, is concentrated fat offering a high cholesterol potential. Whether eaten cooked or uncooked, the fat in the cheese abnormally increases the cholesterol.

Could it be that our God who never changes meant what He said in Leviticus 3:17, "It shall be a perpetual statute for your generations throughout all your dwellings, that ye eat neither fat nor blood"? Dr. Burkitt warns that "even after you have cut the visible fat off your meat, 30 percent even of the lean part can be fat." So he advises "enormously cutting down your meat."

HDL and Good Cholesterol

Then there is *high-density lipoprotein* (HDL), a happy contrast to its dangerous neighbor LDL. Your children might like to think of them as *H*ealthful, *D*elightful *L*ollipops down inside that make their dispositions sweet. HDL helps remove cholesterol from circulation by taking it back to the liver, thus reducing the risk of heart disease.

Weimar allergist Sang Lee says HDL is increased by exercise and happiness. Others add: by laughter and smiles.[3] You can develop HDL by being trustful and faith-filled; by singing happily, listening to inspirational music, cultivating a happy spirit in general, doing things for others and being at peace with the world. You will also find one of its greatest recipes in Isaiah 26:3: "Thou wilt keep him in perfect peace whose mind is stayed on thee, because he trusteth in thee."

Remember also the word, "endorphin," that good little hormone "elf" that is produced by those positive attitudes which help to raise HDL. Such feelings as anger, revenge, hate, envy, evil surmising, competition, and stress have the opposite effect, destroying those precious little elves that work so hard to build your *H*appy *D*elightful *L*ollipops down inside you.

Figuring Your Risks

Another way to figure your risk of coronary heart disease is by ratio: Divide your cholesterol figure by your HDL figure. If the ratio is 4 or less, there is low risk; if 4 to 5, risk is average; at 5 to 6, it is high; at 6–7, it is very high. Figured this way, at the end of four months Dorothy's score had dropped from 7.35 to 4.8 and finally down to 2.47 (166 divided by 67) or less than half the average risk of arteriosclerosis (hardening of the arteries).

A controversy has been going on for years among scientists about the possibility that polyunsaturated fats of vegetable origin, though refined, would lower the level of LDL. Dr. Crane of Weimar Institute points out that in America "most nutritionists have no trouble recognizing the deleterious effects of refined sugar and refined cereals. Yet," he adds sadly, "this concern does not seem to extend to the refined fats." We are forced to take the position with Dr. Crane that refined or "visible" vegetable oils also may have a negative effect. We do this for several reasons:

(1) *Visible* vegetable fats, though unsaturated, include cooking oils, shortening, and margarine, and are prominently contained in mayonnaise and salad dressings. They are made up of refined oils, the process of which is questionable because of the use of either high temperatures or chemicals. Even if the cold-press method is used, common sense should help us understand that the Creator had a good reason to put the elements we need all neatly packaged together in fiber envelopes—natural foods—to provide good nourishment. So let's keep visible fats as low as practical.

When you look at the process and what it does to good food, it makes no more sense to refine fats than it does to refine sugars or to use processed grains. For example, *it takes two pounds of corn to make one ounce of corn oil.* In this wasteful process are refined away most of the vitamins, minerals, 1 ½ pounds of cornstarch, two ounces of protein and ¼ pound of fiber, so that your body must be robbed or deprived of these elements, crippling your metabolism—the turning of your food into flesh and bones and blood and energy.

(2) Visible fat coats the other food used with it—either on the stove or in the stomach—preventing the digestive agent, *ptyalin* from acting efficiently on the starch, and the gastric juices from effectively acting on the protein. Since the digestive process is slowed, the food lies longer in the stomach and putrefies. When it finally reaches the bile duct, the oil is emulsified off and the pancreatic juice digests this decayed food, filling the blood with impurities.

(3) Probably the best proofs for the desirability of a truly natural diet without any refined foods at all, are the miracles that happen in people's lives when they are placed on a diet free from anything but the food elements that are in fruits, grains, nuts, and vegetables. At Weimar, at Hartland Institute and at Uchee Pines, patients whose heart pains are so great they cannot walk across the room, will be seen joyfully walking miles after three or four weeks of lifestyle change. Some have already had heart bypass surgery, and nothing further could be done by their physicians. Others had been scheduled for bypasses who found after such natural treatment that they no longer needed surgery. Such a lifestyle helps the body to clear its own blood channels. Angina patients, freed of animal proteins and fats, are often cured. A number of these patients are physicians or surgeons themselves.

Reversing Artery Blockages

With the right treatment, and assuming the disease has not gone too far, the body has remarkable restorative power. After a session at Weimar, evangelist Ern Baxter and theologian Walter Martin testify to this with great conviction on radio, television, and in print.

Evidence is accumulating that atherosclerosis (hardening of the arteries) may be reversible. During World War II, those prisoners of war who were on "starvation" diets with very little fat, had little or no atherosclerosis, while their agemates who were not interned showed a high prevalence of the disease.

So much for Fat and his bride, Miss Cholesterol. They are sometimes your friends, but make sure that when you are trusting them, *you* are in control!

6

Protein, The Great Pretender

When you are deciding how much confidence to place in your friends, remember that *protein* may be less grabby than *fat*, but he likes to demand your attention, too. He is a valuable friend within his limitations, but he vastly overrates himself at times.

As children both Dorothy and I were taught that we needed a great deal of protein. We were frequently served red meat, fish or chicken. And, depending on the economic situation of the times, we alternated meat with beans. During the years of the Great Depression, beans—often cooked with cheese—became our daily staple. Protein was touted almost everywhere as the most important factor in our diets.

We heard this on the radio (no television then), read it in the papers, were taught it in chemistry and home economics classes, were persuaded by dairy and meat processors' ads, and even learned of it in church. No wonder Americans are obsessed with the idea that they need a lot of protein. And indeed protein is important for health. In some respects it is the key "building material" for our bodies. However, some careful health educators estimate that the average American eats two to four times too much, and the protein excess is undermining our health.

Less Is Better

A number of years ago it was thought that 100 to 150 grams of protein a day were needed. But as different cultures of the world were investigated and found to be doing better on less protein, nutritionists decided that 70 grams a day was sufficient. The more they studied, the more they were convinced our protein rations should be even less.

Now, even though it listens closely to vested interests from the meat and dairy industry, the Food and Nutrition Board of the National Research Foundation of the National Academy of Sciences is recommending only 52–56 grams a day for men, 44–48 grams for women, and 23–26 grams for children. From the best information we can gather, most of us would do well if our protein intake were about 10 percent of the calories we consume. This recommended daily allowance (RDA) makes sense when you realize that it then will not be the same for everybody, for our amount of overall consumption will vary. We will also tell you why it is dangerous to overindulge and why it is great to be in balance. See Chapter 5 on "Reading Labels."

How Much?

The best way to assure yourself that you are getting adequate protein—and not too much—is to eat a variety of properly but simply prepared fruits, grains, nuts (sparingly), and vegetables in quantities sufficient to supply total calories to maintain your proper weight.

We by no means suggest you paralyze yourself with fears that you will not have your calories right on the button. But if you are one of those people who likes to get technical, decide on the number of calories you really need, take 10 percent of that, and then divide by 4 since one gram of protein represents 4 calories. If, as a sedentary worker, you consume 1600 calories a day to maintain your ideal weight, 160 (10 percent) of them should be protein. This 160 divided by 4 tells you that you should be including about 40 grams of protein a day in your diet. While hard physical workers need more, if you are an "easy-keeper" like Dorothy, who does not need so many calories, you may need less.

Though eating too much protein is one of our greatest nutritional faults, not much is told us about what the problems are. A high protein, low carbohydrate diet is still a popular and often-recommended program for weight loss. The reason you need to know the truth is that the results of your protein excesses may not be immediately noticeable. Yet they nevertheless are inevitable, and will be avoided by thoughtful, responsible people when they learn the consequences.

Why Less Protein

In studying this unbalanced diet, Harold Yacowitz and his colleagues at Fairleigh Dickinson University found that a high-protein diet breaks down some protein tissues and causes a *calcium loss* from bone.[1] The result of this is *osteoporosis*, now so widely feared, and periodontal (dental) disease—which we should perhaps fear much more. This condition most commonly involves post-menopausal women.[2] See more in the Addendum of this book.

Such losses of calcium usually are incurred by excretion through the urine, disrupting the *calcium balance*. If the body is not able to absorb enough calcium daily, the blood takes it from bone tissue which is your calcium bank. Eventually, you will have weak, demineralized bones.[3]

Calcium loss is said to afflict as many as 20,000,000 Americans. At least 1,300,000 fractures are attributed to this affliction; 20 percent of these die of complications and another 20 percent become permanently crippled. The "dowager's hump"—compression of the vertebrae with accompanying loss of height—and other bone problems are also symptoms of this bone deterioration.

Drs. Calvin and Agatha Thrash of the Medical Board for this book point out that "there is a 1.4% annual loss of bone calcium after age 50 in women who take even one cup of coffee daily, or 14% loss per decade!" Smoking and drinking as well as excessive coffee drinking are also implicated in bone calcium loss.[4]

Calcium loss is one of a number of ways a high protein diet *accelerates the aging process*.[5] To be fair, it should also be noted that the commonly decreased physical activity—lack of exercise—and declining estrogen levels of these women play a part in contributing to the problem.[6]

Vegetarian Advantages

However, bone deterioration has been shown to be much less prevalent among women who are lacto-ovo-vegetarians (those who eat eggs and milk but no meat). In a research study of women 50–89 years of age, the vegetarian women lost only half as much bone mineral mass as the nonvegetarian women.[7] Dorothy was one of the subjects of that study.

The Thrashes, in their editing of this book, also stated that in all their extensive clinical work they have yet to see an unexpected fracture in elderly people who are pure vegetarians, even though most of them are quite thin.

Animal protein seems to put higher stress on the body than vegetable protein. It produces, among other things, excessive amounts of sulfur-containing amino acids that break down into sulfates, which in turn cause reduced reabsorption of calcium into the blood. Then more calcium appears in the urine.[8] On the other hand, legumes—peas, beans, lentils, and so on—which provide plant food protein, are low in these sulfur-containing amino acids, and help to account for less calcium loss among the vegetarian women.

Ridding Excesses

High protein puts a heavy burden on the kidneys by increasing the rate of filtration and an increased blood flow. Even the reserve filtering units in the kidneys are compelled to be in almost constant usage which causes them to progressively harden and bring about eventual deterioration of kidney function.[9]

Still another risk of a high animal protein diet is the possibility of developing kidney stones—which are largely composed of calcium salts.[10]

Obviously God designed the chemistry of the human body so that when you live according to His plan, your system takes care of your needs efficiently, barring accidents or infectious disease. When treated properly, your body will discard what is excess. In one experiment subjects were fed a diet with *normal* amounts of all nutrients including calcium. They retained an average of 375 mg. of calcium per day during the experiment. On the other hand, a matched group which received a *high* calcium diet retained only 103 mg. of calcium per day![11]

Dangerous Losses

In another study to determine the effect of protein intake on calcium loss, three groups of participants consumed 1400 mg. (1.4 grams) of calcium a day, but varied their amounts of protein intake with dramatic differences in calcium gain: Those who ate 48 grams of protein a day averaged a calcium *gain* of 20 points on a set scale. Those who ate 95 grams of protein a day had a *loss* of 25 points! Those who ate 142 grams of protein a day suffered an astonishing calcium *loss*.[12] Indeed, *it has been found that a high calcium diet will likely not compensate for such calcium losses resulting from high protein diets![13]*

This close relationship between the amount of protein consumed and the calcium needs of the body brings us to the ideal amount of calcium a day which we should include. The National Academy of Sciences' Food and Nutrition Board have set 800 milligrams per day as the "recommended daily allowance" (RDA) for Americans. At the time this was discussed at length by the Board it was found that *if* the RDA of protein was kept at the proper level, 500 mg. per day would be adequate. Some nutritionists even believed 350 mg. should be adequate, but the rationale for the higher U.S. figures, as reported by *Nutrition Today* (Mar/Apr 1974, pp. 20 and 21) is the high protein intakes prevalent in the U.S. This is considerably higher than the amount of calcium recommended in Canada, the United Kingdom, and by the World Health Organization.

In other words, since we consume so much animal protein, we better do the best we can about trying to compensate for the great calcium loss it causes. As you have already seen, the real solution lies in a more "prudent" diet which utilizes calcium more fully and less is excreted.

Supplying Calcium

Calcium needs are not so great but that they can be easily supplied from totally vegetable sources. All plant foods contain calcium in varying amounts. But for an especially plentiful supply, eat plenty of broccoli (one cup contains 206 mg. of calcium); one cup of

Food Facts

	Edible Calories per 100 Grams (3–½ oz.)	Calcium mg	Protein %	Fat %	Carbohyd. %
FRUITS					
Apples (⅔ medium)	58	6.3	1.2	8.7	90.1
Avocados (⅔ c. cubed or scant ½ c. puree)	167	8.8	4.2	82.2	13.6
Bananas (½ banana)	85	5.5	4.3	2.0	93.7
Blueberries (½ c.)	62	15.5	3.8	6.9	89.3
Carob (¾ c.)	180	296.0	8.4	6.5	85.0
Dates (12 dates)	275	58.7	2.7	1.5	95.8
Grapefruit (¼)	41	4.5	4.1	2.0	93.9
Grapes (20 seedless)	69	12.6	6.4	12.1	81.5
Oranges (½ c. diced)	49	40.0	7.0	3.4	89.6
Peaches (1 small peach or ½ large)	39	7.8	5.3	2.2	92.5
Tomatoes (1 tomato, 2⅗" dia.)	22	12.0	12.3	7.7	76.4
GRAINS					
Cornmeal (whole ground, ¾ c.)	355	19.6	7.1	9.2	83.7
Millet (1 cup)	327	20.1	12.1	7.8	69.0
Rice, Brown (½ c. dry)	360	32.0	7.1	4.4	88.5
Rolled Oats, dry (1 cup)	390	52.5	12.6	15.9	71.5
Wheat (whole ground, ¾ c.)	330	15.0	13.3	4.6	82.1
Wheat (shredded, flakes, 3⅓ c.)	354	40.0	10.0	4.7	85.3
LEGUMES					
Beans (pinto, dried, ½ c.)	349	135.0	22.8	2.9	74.3
Garbanzos (dried, ½ c.)	360	150.0	19.8	11.2	69.0
Lentils (dried, ½ c.)	340	79.0	25.3	2.7	72.0
Peanuts (¾ c. shelled, chopped.)	582	74.0	15.6	70.0	14.4
Peas (⅝ c. cooked)	84	23.0	26.1	4.0	69.9
Soybeans, cooked (⅔ cup)	134	72.0	28.2	31.8	40.0
Tofu (⅔ cup)	77	128.0	38.0	51.0	11.0
NUTS AND SEEDS					
Almonds (¾ c. raw whole)	598	233.0	10.8	75.9	13.3
Coconut (dried, 3½ oz.)	662	26.0	3.8	82.1	14.1
Sunflower (dried, scant ¾ c.)	560	120.0	14.9	70.6	14.5
Walnuts (1 c. halves)	628	119.0	11.3	79.1	9.6
Cashews (3½ oz. or ¾ c. whole)	561	38.0	17.2	48.7	29.3
VEGETABLES					
Asparagus (4 large cooked spears)	26	21.0	23.5	6.4	68.9
Beans, green (¾ c. cooked)	32	50.4	14.5	5.3	80.0
Beets, raw (¾ c. diced)	43	16.2	10.2	1.9	88.4
Broccoli (⅔ c. chopped, cooked)	32	90.6	27.5	7.8	65.9
Carrots (1 c. grated raw)	42	40.0	7.4	4.0	88.8
Celery (6 small inner stalks)	17	40.0	12.9	4.9	81.8
Cucumbers (1 c. chopped)	15	26.0	14.7	5.6	80.7
Onions (1 c. sliced)	38	30.0	11.0	2.2	87.8
Parsley (1–1¼ c. chopped)	44	207.0	20.0	11.4	68.9
Potatoes (½ baked)	76	7.0	7.6	1.1	90.7
MEATS, POULTRY (¼ lb. approx.)					
Hamburger (lean, raw)	179	48.0	49.9	50.1	-0-
Sirloin (choice, broiled)	387	11.0	25.4	74.6	-0-
Chicken (light, roasted)	166	10.0	81.5	18.5	-0-
Leg of lamb (roasted)	319	7.9	32.1	67.9	-0-
Pork loin (roasted)	362	12.0	28.9	71.1	-0-
FISH					
Tuna (canned, oil drained, ⅝ c.)	197	8.0	62.5	37.5	-0-
Tuna (canned, water—not drained, ½ cup)	127	16.0	94.2	5.8	-0-
EGGS, MILK					
Eggs, poached (1 egg—approx 50 gm)	163	26.0	34.0	64.2	1.8
Milk, whole (3.5% fat) (⅓ cup approx.)	65	117.0	23.0	47.6	29.4
Milk, skimmed (⅓ c. approx.)	36	128.0	42.8	2.5	54.7
CHEESES					
Cheese, cheddar (1 c. approx.)	398	750.0	26.8	71.1	2.1
Parmesan, hard (4 T. approx.)	393	1200.0	39.1	58.1	2.8

Source:

Edible calories per 100 grams—from data in U.S. Dept. of Agriculture Handbook #8, Table 1.

Percent of total calories of protein, fat and carbohydrate: computed from data in U.S. Dept of Agriculture Handbook #8, Tables 1 and 6.

All figures given are for uncooked foods, unless specifically mentioned as cooked.

almost any cooked greens—including collards, mustard, turnips, kale, dandelions, lambsquarters or brussel sprouts and legumes are a good source. Two tablespoons of whole sesame seeds give you about 258 mg.

Other Dietary Cautions

High protein may cause possible damage to the immune system through incomplete digestion. Reasons for the harm these may do are explained in a variety of other places. (See index and also the chapter on Dairy Products for macromolecules and infant allergies.)

You should also be cautious not to eat soon after violent or heavy exercise or when you are excited, anxious, hurried or even if you are worried, angry or resentful. These emotions disturb the proper function of the blood supply through the digestive system. A merry heart is really better than a medicine!

I am well-acquainted with a widow whose husband was a high-strung individual whom she dearly loved and missed greatly as long as she lived. She never realized why her colitis, nervous indigestion, and catarrh (all largely emotionally caused problems) completely disappeared after he died. She discovered that she could eat "almost anything, even onions, without any distress!"

Easy-to-get Protein

"But however do you get enough protein?" This is the most frequent question vegetarians are asked. Yet the answer is really simple, because all growing things contain protein and it's easier to get too much than too little, especially if you also eat milk and eggs. Legumes, meaning all the varieties of beans, peas, lentils, and garbanzos offer a bonus in the plentiful amount of iron which

COMPARE

COMPARISON OF FREE FATS AND NUTS					
	Calories	Calcium mg	Protein gms	Fats gms	Carb. gms
Corn oil—1 Cup	1927			218	
Shelled almonds—1 Cup	849	332	26.4	77	27.7
Walnuts, shelled—1 Cup	785		25.6	74	18.5
Cashews, shelled—1 Cup	675	53	24.1	54	41.0

From WEIMAR INSTITUTE, WEIMAR CA, 1985

they also supply. Soybeans have an especially high count and give you plenty of calcium (146 mg. in one cup, cooked) and riboflavin besides. Some nutritionists advise using legumes four or five times a week. See Food Facts chart on page 60.

The myth that plant food may not be able to supply quality (or "complete") protein has also been long set aside by studies which show that a mixture of plant proteins has a comparable quality to animal proteins and in some instances is superior. Of the four plant sources of protein (legumes, nuts, grains, and seeds), a mixture of any will yield a complete protein.

In case you don't eat a "complete" protein at one meal, you still don't have to worry. An amino acid pool forms in the bloodstream and tissue, stored from the food you eat. Then when the right amino acids come along from the next meal they combine with the ones already there to make up a complete protein! And all the essential amino acids in adequate amounts will be found in such a meal.[14]

7

Milk: For Kids or for Calves?

Questioning the wisdom of using dairy products may seem almost un-American to some. While coffee comes to us largely from overseas, milk has been the great American drink—aided and abetted, of course, by the dairy industry which at one time would not allow any butter substitutes, not even margarine. In the United States, each of us consumes an average of 385 pounds of dairy products a year.

Milk is a source of high-quality protein, and is rich with calcium, phosphorus, and Vitamin B 12.[1] Yet each animal is endowed with milk of a unique quality for its own young. This does not mean that the milk of one beast will never do for another, but there is evidence enough that the Creator knew what He was doing when He designed each creature. And there is also good reason to believe that He designed milk as a food for infants, not adults, much as we hate to have to admit it here, for we have long been milk "fans" (short for *fanatics*).

That Unique Mother's Milk

The wisdom of using any other milk except that made especially for babies (mother's milk) is now being questioned. Each mammal has a different composition of milk for its young, and only mother's

63

milk is ideal for the human infant, according to many scientists. In comparing the fine, flaky, easily digestible curds of mother's milk with that of a cow—''which has curds the size of the end of your finger''—Dr. Harry Miller, the great ''China Doctor,'' always insisted that cow's milk was designed with calves in mind.[2]

Cautions on Cows' Milk

The evidence is mounting that milk and milk products are linked to a number of health problems. One is iron-deficiency anemia in 15 to 20 percent of children under the age of two. Milk is low in iron, containing less than 1 mg of iron per quart, very little of which is absorbed because of other constituents of the milk. It also may induce gastrointestinal bleeding in sensitive infants, causing a loss of 1 to 5 milliliters of blood per day.[3]

Cow's milk contains three basic ingredients—sugar, fat, and protein, two of which have already been cited as problems in nutrition. *Lactase* which breaks down *lactose,* the sugar component in milk and milk products, is found in the intestinal cells of the upper part of the gastrointestinal tract and is concentrated in that part of the small bowel called the jejunum.[4] Lactase activity in the fetus begins during the last third of pregnancy, is at its height shortly after birth, and decreases sometime between the ages of 1 ½ and four years in 60 percent to 75 percent of individuals. This process, which occurs in most mammals shortly after they are weaned, has caused many scientists to conclude that no one should drink milk after he is weaned.

Investigators at the Johns Hopkins School of Medicine first observed in 1965 that 15 percent of whites and 70 percent of all blacks tested were unable to digest lactose. The majority of people in this world, mostly black or yellow, are ''lactose intolerant.''[5] In the cells that line the intestines of the normal infant, the enzyme lactase splits the lactose apart into glucose and galactose. Some youngsters lose their ability to make lactase enzyme about age 4, and their lactose goes undigested. Although this is not a food allergy, its reactions similarly may come, for example, as indigestion, nausea, and diarrhea.[6]

You may remember the problems created by the U.S. shipment of powdered milk to South American countries before this lactase deficiency was discovered. The natives carefully reconstituted the milk with water, but after it was used, cramps and diarrhea broke out in the villages. The conclusion was that it was another "imperialist plot." It seems that next time they diluted the powder with less water and used it to whitewash their huts. Dr. Frank A. Oski, the author of a book called *Don't Drink Your Milk,*[7] comments that "some American scientists believe the U.S. dairy industry has been attempting to whitewash" the problem ever since.

Those Special Molecules

Absorption of macromolecules—oversized molecules—is the source of the difficulty you often hear about when infants are allergic to cow's milk. It can even develop when the mother has *used* cow's milk during her pregnancy. During the first eighteen months of life, the infant has an increased capacity to ingest certain macromolecules without a problem. Milk proteins were designed in a molecular shape which would allow them to go through special nonselective sites in the intestinal wall to supply antibodies from mother to young. These special sites may later on permit the big molecules from cow's milk and other foods to be absorbed (bear in mind again that each animal's milk has its own makeup of protein, fat, and minerals).[8]

This molecular movement apparently was the Creator's plan to allow globulin *antibodies* to be transferred from the mother's breast milk to the infant—an important component to help guarantee baby's immediate and future health. In other words, mother's milk provides important immunities. It is unlikely that cow's milk or even soy milk was ever intended as a substitute for human milk, because of the crossing of these "foreign" macromolecules through the intestinal wall where, as we have noted, they are likely to create distress. This includes also the possibility that they may induce colic and allergy problems. If you want the best opportunities for your new baby, you might do well to cut back or to omit cow's milk during your pregnancy.[9]

Infant Allergies

Multiple forms of allergy in infants have been estimated to range as high as 25 percent. Symptoms may be persistent or recurring respiratory (nasal and bronchial) congestion, skin rash, vomiting or diarrhea which cannot be explained otherwise. A study of 787 babies under one year of age, personally supervised by Dr. J. W. Gerrard and his associates in Canada, disclosed 7.5 percent allergic to cow's milk. Twenty-five percent of those fed cow's milk before three months of age showed some signs of allergy, indicating that the earlier in the child's life that he was given cow's milk, the more likely he was to show allergic symptoms.[10]

Milk-transmitted Diseases

Though pasteurization of milk is a safety measure to guard against the spread of disease germs, it does not destroy bacillus which causes listerosis—a disease affecting animals, birds, and occasionally man, which brings fever and paralysis.[11] It is doubtful that cancer viruses are destroyed by pasteurization either. Cancer viruses of leukemia and other sorts are known to be transmitted from one animal to another through milk. Another disease carried by milk is streptococcus.[12]

We now know that diseases of many kinds, including cancer viruses of leukemia and other types, can be transmitted from one animal to the next through milk.[13] A cow may have leukemia for months before she is sick enough to be taken out of the herd. Meanwhile she may not only have infected other cattle, but also transmitted cancer viruses into her milk for human consumption. The only certain way to be sure that such viruses are dead is to boil the milk for at least ten minutes. Pasteurization, as we have noted, is not enough.[14]

Beyond these problems are, of course, the dangers of drugs and antibiotics administered to cattle who are sick, but not sick enough to be taken from the herd. Thus resistance may be built up in the human body, upon drinking their milk. Or, people may develop allergies even after infancy.

Those Delicious Cheeses

Cheese, long a favorite food of ours, and considered by many vegetarians to be a good meat substitute, may in some of its forms and for some people be one of the most unwholesome foods of all. In the first place, it is most often coagulated by rennet made from finely ground calves' stomachs or pepsin from innards of swine—although a few cheesemakers claim that they do not use animal enzymes.[15]

Dr. Mervyn Hardinge, a physician who is also a Harvard-trained public health doctor and a Stanford-educated pharmacologist, has made a study of cheeses from medical and nutritional points of view. He notes that "only a few cheeses are sold *fresh* or *unripened*, usually using a lactic starter (although sometimes adding rennet or pepsin): cottage cheese, cream cheese, pot cheese, fresh Neufchatel and Ricotta."[16] The U.S. Department of Agriculture divides cheeses into three groups: *hard* (cheddar or "American"); *semihard* (brick and rocquefort), and *soft* (Limburger and Camembert). All of these are ripened by bacteria except rocquefort and Camembert, in which penicillin mold is used.[17]

Wholesome Cheese?

Bacteria and molds work on the proteins, fats, and carbohydrates of the curd through a process of fermentation and decomposition. The older and sharper cheeses come from longer processing.

While some organisms are beneficial to man, there are serious questions about the wholesomeness of cheeses developed by rennet, pepsin, bacteria or molds.[18]

Tyramine, a substance found abundantly in cheddar cheese, beer, and some wines, often brings on migraine headaches. It is not alone, however, for such foods as milk, chocolate, wheat, and pork have also been suspected. While mental mechanisms may trigger migraine, the person who falls prey most easily is likely to be the one who eats tyramine-related foods.[19]

It is well known, of course, that cheese offers a certain cholesterol risk in combination with animal fats. Hypertension patients must usually avoid cheeses as well as salt, sugar, red meats, and coffee.

Un-American or not, you may find it to your welfare and the health of your family to reexamine the place of dairy products in your diet. We do not suggest that you be in a hurry. There is no need to panic. But with both research and common sense asking some valid questions, you may want to look again.

. . . present your bodies a living sacrifice . . .

Romans 12:1

8

Those Vege Nuts

"I never, ever, thought of it that way!" A prominent evangelical was shaking his head on the occasion when we were leaving one of Bill Gothard's family counseling seminars to go with him and his staff to lunch.

A companion agreed: "It takes some courage, but it's not going to make him popular with some theologians!"

Bill had just given his new lecture on clean and unclean meats which pointed to modern scientific backing for the Mosaic restrictions on eating certain fish, fowl, and animals.

"Yet, if that is true, and God means what He says," the first reasoned out loud, "if we're really planning on living in heaven, we should be eating as much like heaven as we can down here."

"You're talking like a *vege nut,*" chided the other.

Not for Christians Only

I remembered someone writing recently that everything that the Christian does is done with eternity in mind. Only thus will our *death* style become a *life* style, a *living sacrifice.* Some consider this a Judeo-Christian ethic, but orthodox Jews tend to be much more conservative on this subject than Christians. Muslims also have more than a little of this bent in their thinking. They tend to be much more disciplined than Christians. Even Hindus are alert to their Nirvana and dietary readiness. Anyway, several "veges" were born that day, although that was not Bill's announced goal. And many more are moving in this direction.

But for most vegetarians other reasons have long reigned. At first we had some hesitation about laying them out here. Some, we reasoned, would think we had a fetish. And it was almost certain that meat eaters will not understand—and may be disappointed—that vege nuts do not feel deprived at all. Nearly all of them delight in their nuttiness.

Our editors answered without batting an eye, "Tell it like it is. You give them good information, and let them make up their own minds." So we tell you just a few of the *whys* of vegetarianism without accusing you of sin if you don't agree. Yet it represents only a small part of a great persuasive picture:

Why Vegetarian?

For some, the idea of killing any living thing unnecessarily for food is an unpleasant thought. For some, like us, the first questions, or the vegetarian resolve, came with a visit to a slaughterhouse or the back of a butcher shop. Others fear disease. For yet others, particularly Jews, the taste of meat that has met orthodox standards isn't this great. And there are of course many around the world who are vegetarians out of necessity or because they are economy minded, and vegetables cost less.

The concept of the heavenly diet is an overriding reason for many, for it pretty well includes the others. The ecologist who considers himself too humane to kill and eat is also seeing his tribe increase. But those groups concerned about disease probably account for the most rapid growth of vegetarianism these days, and from substantial evidence. Diseases of animals are transmitted to man mostly by the blood.

Eating Animal Waste

No wonder that Gentiles are usually disappointed when they first try kosher meats. At least that was our experience. The taste of the meat is heightened usually in proportion to the amount of blood and the tang that uric acid gives it, particularly in the red meats. I remember that, as a long-distance truck driver, I knew which truck stops had the juiciest hot roast beef sandwiches. And then one day I was married, and my bride told me something about what was in the blood, and why God warned Old Testament Israel not to eat fat or blood.

The uric acid in the animal's blood is a waste product—the stuff of which urine is made. Urine in the animal's body is converted to uric acid, urea, and ammonia. All these nitrogen-containing compounds build up in the blood, and after you eat a flesh meal will begin to show up in increasing amounts in *your* urine![1]

Although the idea of eating for one's heaven is much more lofty, the distasteful notion of eating the animal's waste—combined with almost certain exposure to disease—turned me into a vegetarian overnight. I decided that vege nuts have a lot of logic going for them.

Take one simple experience that has been repeated in my life many times. As the vice-president of a university which had a major medical school, I found that members of our staff were often hassled by well-meaning folks who insisted that we should never use animals for experimentation. For some, just to remind them of the origin of vaccines and other preventatives and remedies, was enough to help them rethink their protests. But the most poignant question in the staff's quiver was, "Are you a vegetarian?" If they were not, that settled it. Vegetarians are the only activists who can with any logic protest the use of animals in research. All others *eat* them.

"Approving" the Flesh Diet

Noah and the Ark generally provide a landmark for the meat eater. After the Great Flood when the lush vegetation of Eden was gone and the earth had not fully revegetated itself, the Bible tells us that God gave Noah and his family a right He had not previously granted: "Everything that lives and moves will be food for you. Just as I gave you the green plants, I now give you everything." And then He added, hardly as an afterthought, "But you must not eat meat that has its lifeblood still in it."[2] Even then the lifespan of man dropped from over 900, down to about 120 years.

Disease

As the world became more degenerate and diseased, and the human race became weaker, God, through Moses, saw fit to restrict the Israelites—His chosen people—to "clean" meats.[3] He insisted that they eat only the food of animals which both chewed the cud and had cloven hoofs. So while cows and sheep were approved, for example, pigs, rabbits, and frogs were not. The Mosaic instructions specified that edible fish must have both fins and scales, so catfish, oysters, shrimp, and crabs were not to be eaten. Unclean fowl were explicitly proscribed by name, such as hawks, owls, vultures, ravens, storks, and herons.

Changing Conditions: Fish and Fowl

Disease and degeneracy had taken their toll, so that by King David's time[4] the normal lifespan was down to "three score and ten"—where it generally lingers today. I once argued that if Christ ate fish, so can I. And I can. Yet I was forced to face an increase in disease so great that as many as 60 to 100 percent of some kinds of fish in American lakes and streams are cancerous.[5] In ocean fish, statistics are no better. Over 50 percent of two-year-old codfish are cancerous.

Over the last 50 to 75 years the dumping of raw or partially treated sewage into inland and coastal waters has almost certainly contributed to this dangerous and devastating condition. This has been documented in countless studies. A Smithsonian Institution investigation of such waters in North America pinpoints danger zones from Puget Sound, Washington, Yaquina Bay, Oregon, Santa Ana, California and the Gulf of California, through states of the Great Lakes to Alabama, and to the East Coast from Maine to the Florida Keys.[6] It was found that when coho salmon from the Great Lakes was fed to laboratory rats, the little animals developed the same diseases as the fish.[7]

Dr. Richard Adamson, Director of Cancer Cause and Prevention at the National Cancer Institute was asked about the Great Lakes findings. While he would not yet make definitive scientific conclusions, he did have his own private opinions: "I would not eat any fish that I knew came from those areas."[8]

Specialists at the U.S. Department of Agriculture in Maryland recently confirmed to us by telephone what they said "all animal specialists know," namely that nearly all chickens are infected with some form of leukosis or other disease, and their only salvation as a food lies in their vaccination for these maladies. Hundreds of millions of pounds of poultry are yearly condemned by food inspectors, and many millions of pounds of beef, mutton, swine, and so on.[9] Federal inspectors, careful as they are, are hardly able to account for a much larger number of diseased animals, fish, and fowl that are passed over.

Meat Inspection

Even the hundreds of millions of pounds of animals condemned are small figures compared with the number of those passed. The question repeatedly raised by the Amalgamated Butchers Union of America and other agencies has been, "How many do the Federal meat inspectors miss?" Some union officials believe that with budgetary limitations and the pressures of many diseases, a large number are missed. Some physicians and health specialists are convinced that the rise in leukemia among children, for example, is directly related to the high incidence of this disease in chickens.

If the inspectors don't see it, no matter how diseased the animal is, they don't call it. Gordon H. Theilen, D.V.M., of the University of California Agricultural Experiment Station, speaking of leukemia in *cattle,* confirmed that while it "is easy for meat inspectors to identify the terminal clinical form. . . . *the microscopic leukemic stage will be missed every time if there is no gross enlargement, since blood studies are not conducted before slaughter.*"[10]

Veges Have It

As we write this, in the spring of 1986, we receive the current issue of the Tufts University *Diet and Nutrition Letter*[11] in which the editors address the very concerns we express here.

If the proof of the "pudding"[12] is in the eating, the veges have it, for they live with less disease and, at age 40, live at least six or seven years older, on the average, than do carnivorous human beings. Still we should point out that there are areas where fresh fruits and vegetables are hard to come by. In such event, for example in remote areas of Alaska, a dinner of salmon or moose might be the better part of both wisdom and valor.

First Corinthians 10:31 admonishes us to eat and drink "to the glory of God." To us this means "Eat the best available food," and to study how we can do even better and be approved unto God. Some other religions appear to adopt even firmer resolves than Christians do in general. Many Muslims would die before they would eat pork.

Then why should Americans be among the greatest consumers of red meats in the world? Editor Jack Pickett of the *California Farmer* wrote me a few years ago that ". . . most people, as they become affluent, have shown an increased desire for red meats."[13] Mr. Pickett added that "The depth of this desire was startling to the experts and now we see the same latent hunger in developing countries."

Rampant Cattle Disease

Some years ago the USDA reported that 35 percent of cattle and swine slaughtered in this country are not subjected to Federal inspection.[14] Recently a New York City butcher remarked to some of us that he would not allow his family to touch meat. He observed that the "disease is so bad [pervasive] that they only cut out the largest tumors." Lest this sound like a fanatic who was trying to make some veges feel good, I quote the Consumers Union report of several years ago that "A shockingly large percentage of the hamburger we purchased was well on the way to putrefaction."[15]

Unclean Meats

Obviously inspectors cannot do fine checks, for example on trichinae in pork—which admittedly afflict tens of millions of Americans. Most of the victims of these little worms attribute their aches and pains to other causes, unaware that the *trichinella spiralis*, a tiny wormlike parasite, has pierced the lining of their intestines and finally lodged most likely in the muscles of the diaphragm and legs. Some estimates suggest that at least 15 to 20 percent of all Americans suffer with this gift from pork, which sometimes brings another gift—death. This may help to understand why the Mosaic instructions forbade swine as food for Old Testament Israel.

Likewise catfish—with fins, but no scales—was thought to be a safe food, despite Mosaic injunctions. But certain Bible doubters had to do some rethinking when catfish was found to be a principal source of erysipelas: Its victims suffer from feverish inflammation of the skin and mucuous membrane which often affect the membranes which line the cavities of the heart, or result in septicemia—serious infections in the bloodstream, and various forms of arthritis. Some fish, such as swordfish, may contain nerve toxins.

Money

The least obvious reason for changing diets may in time become the leading one: money. To match quality of vegetarian diets with those centered on flesh will usually bring the carrot-chewers well out ahead, unless for example, you make your living fishing for salmon off Kodiak. Just how much difference surprised even us a few years ago. *Today's Health* pointed out that a man's protein requirements for less than 250 days required the meat of animals fed from one acre of land. But the same acre sown in grains— wheat, rice, corn—will provide enough protein for 527 to 773 days. An acre of soybeans raises the ante to 2200 days. When costed out, the magazine found that one pound of beef-derived protein then cost $4.44, while a pound of soy protein then cost 11 cents.

Ever-present Disease

You may subconsciously think, *It surely won't happen to me.* And it may not. But increasingly disease *is* taking its toll. A trip to a few oncology wards in general hospitals may give you a more persuasive picture of death styles than we can do here. Yet whether you have a humanitarian concern for animals, or fear of disease or a desire to save money, the truth about flesh eating is as scientifically based as that of smoking and chewing tobacco, drinking alcohol, and going on drugs.

Addendum

As an addendum to this chapter, we offer the comments of Drs. Bernell and Marjorie Baldwin, he a neurophysiologist and she a physician, on some of their trips to a Southern California slaughter-house. This is not pleasant reading, so you may want to skip the remainder of this chapter, except for the last two paragraphs. These scientists provide a forthright report of the scenes which the conscientious food inspector has to face daily:

The animals are brought in large cattle trucks and discharged into fenced holding pens where they are kept for up to three days. They are fed, and water is available. Some of the cows were still fresh—udders heavy with milk, often dripping. Inflamed teats and udders, probably indicating mastitis, were in evidence. . . . There were two cows with eye growths that the veterinarian diagnosed as "epithelioma of the eye"—a very common cancer in cattle. One young steer had a distorted face, with a prominent bulge above his nose. Actinomycosis, thought Dr. Inspector. A number had swollen, apparently painful joints, probably arthritis.

On another visit about two dozen cattle in one pen had "B" branded on their cheeks. Dr. Inspector explained that these had reacted positively to a test for brucellosis, or undulant fever. Two cows, obviously sick, were lying just outside the closest pen. One had obvious mastitis. We took its temperature—104.4 [degrees] F. Our informant said that if the temperature manifested a downward trend, this cow could be used for food. If not, she would be condemned. The other was bleeding from the uterus.

From the closest holding area, the animals walk single file up a narrow ramp at the end of which they pass behind a curtain and are struck in the head. Frequently, sensing disaster ahead, an animal will attempt to turn around. Finding the trail too narrow, it will attempt to back down—sometimes in panic. A long, slender, flexible, electrified prod in the hands of a skillful operator assists in bovine cooperation. We saw the prod inserted into the rectum for special persuasion. These methods cannot but fill the body with stress hormones.

Once felled by a puncturing blow to the head, the cow, now inside the cooled building, is quickly strung up by the legs, and the neck is slit. Blood from all animals gushes into a below-floor-level tank and is then channeled to a waiting truck that carries it away to be processed. When drained of [most of] the blood, the cow is serially processed by butchers in assembly-line style. Head and feet are removed; the skin is slit and removed; abdominal organs are emptied into a cart; head, liver, tongue, and feet are hung on respective racks with dozens of others; and the carcass is swung along on an overhead transport system. . . .

According to *The American Farmer* (January, 1974) suitable feed for beef and cattle and sheep can be made as silage, using 70 percent crop wastes, either chopped cornstalks or oat straw and 30 percent cattle or poultry manure. . . .

Various parasitic diseases . . . are fairly common. These usually do not require condemnation. . . . [Yet parasites] frequently present in food animals are as dangerous to man as they ever were. The cautions sounded for many years and frequently unheeded, that all animal flesh should be thoroughly cooked, is still valid. Animals commonly used for food still harbor tapeworms, and anyone eating raw or rare beef that contained just one live bladderworm (cysticerci) can be infected. [*Animal Diseases*, The Yearbook of Agriculture (1956), U.S. Department of Agriculture, Washington, D.C., p. 22] Other tapeworms, including those of some fresh-water fish, and roundworms, including hookworms, are still common.[16]

The Baldwins go on to document that there is a "direct relationship between intake of animal proteins and deaths from intestinal cancer," including bowel cancer. And this has been known for many years through both professional and popular journals.[17] They warn, among many other dangers, that a flesh diet can negatively affect the immune system, especially in young children.[18] It confuses blood clotting.[19] And it has long been known that it even interferes with the efficient operation of the brain.[20] This apparently depressing effect may in part explain the Scriptures when Israel demanded quail in addition to their heaven-sent manna: "He gave them their request; but sent leanness into their soul" (Psalm 106:15).

Conclusion

So the *quality* of life as well as its length, is at stake when we compare a diet of second-hand food with natural nutrition. There is obviously a much more likely chance of disease in meat diets than there is in those of fruits, grains, nuts, and vegetables. Whether or not we should be pure vegetarians or occasionally use milk, butter, and eggs is part and parcel of other chapters in this book. We do not make judgments here; this diet may not be for everyone. And surely, as we have observed, meat may be the only survival route in some regions. We provide sound scientific and clinical information. Yet, whatever our concern—or lack of it—for health and lifestyle here, there does seem to be more than a little logic, and some spiritual value in eating for the society of heaven.

When you sit to dine with a ruler . . .
do not crave his delicacies.

Proverbs 23:1, 3

9

Spice and Everything "Nice"

For a long time we have heard some not-so-nice things about additives, leaveners, salts, seasonings, spices and supplements, and even some herbs. But I thought they came from sour-grapes people who seemed bent on taking all the joy out of life. After all Dad had set the example for us at home, and he loved spices. We always had lots of cinnamon, sugar, and milk on our rice. We had still more cinnamon in our applesauce, pumpkin pie, cinnamon rolls, and even on cottage cheese. And for more years than I can remember, Dad scattered black pepper all over his fried potatoes and eggs. To us boys that was a sign of manliness, and we sneaked pepper whenever we could.

Then, after Dorothy and I were married, along came some busy bodies and solemnly warned us about eating fresh homemade bread. It had something to do with the action of yeast, and they insisted that fresh-baked, yeast-raised bread should be set aside for at least twenty-four hours. There went my favorite of all taste treats— homemade, hot, oven-fresh bread with lots of butter melted all over it. I protested that at least it was whole wheat, but that didn't placate these joy-killers; in fact, they said that the kind of flour had little to do with the "problem." We found later that it was we who had some lessons to learn!

Common Table Salt

It took Dorothy and me nearly fifty years to become alert to the overuse of *salt*—the common table chemical, sodium chloride. We never were heavy salt users, and have used few condiments, relishes or spices of any kind during our marriage—now forty-eight years. Yet Dorothy is now forced on a salt-free diet because she has hypertension, commonly known as high blood pressure, often with constricting or narrowing of her blood vessels. This can, among other things, damage her arteries, and then her eyes, kidneys, liver, and heart.

And salt is not alone. There are dozens of additives, leavenings, seasonings, spices, and supplements which titillate your taste buds or preserve your foods or raise your biscuits and bread at the expense of your health. Yet we are glad to report that there are some very special extras such as many herbs and harmless, even healthful, seasonings which you may freely deploy in your body.

Salt, of course, is not the only cause of hypertension. Family history, stress, and the wrong dietary fat may be far more to blame among those who suffer from this puzzling "disease." Dorothy may have to take minimal medication the rest of her life for this dangerous annoyance, for doctors still do not know exactly what triggers it in all cases. Yet added salt usually is the first dietary item they eliminate along with insistence on weight reduction.

It is estimated that the average American consumes thirty-five times as much salt as his body needs. The U.S. Senate Select Committee on Nutrition recommends that Americans reduce salt consumption from an average of 15 grams to 5 grams of added salt a day—equivalent to about one teaspoon which contains 2000 milligrams of sodium. The tables given here are not intended to shock you, yet are a warning to ponder.[1]

The comparison of the sodium in processed foods with the same food in its natural form is also enlightening—the amount of sodium in 100 grams, for example, of sweet corn which has only a trace of sodium, equivalent canned corn with 236 milligrams, and corn-flakes with 1005.

When you realize that nearly all processed foods, including most breakfast cereals, are well-salted, it is easy to understand why most of us are oversalted. If and when you decide to lower your intake of this tempting substance, your food will at first seem dull

Not Only from Your Saltshaker

Low	Serving size	Milligrams of Sodium
coffee	1 cup	1
fruit juice	1 cup	2–10
fruit	1	2–5
tea	1 cup	5
broccoli	½ cup	8
tomato	1	14
soft drinks	1 cup	10–60
egg	1	60
beef, pork, lamb, poultry, fish (fresh)	3 ounces	60–100
Medium		
butter, salted	1 tablespoon	115
margarine	1 tablespoon	115
milk	1 cup	120
cake	2 ounces	150–400
ketchup	1 tablespoon	180
bread	2 slices	200–600
shellfish, fresh	3 ounces	200–300
English muffin	1	210
High		
mustard	1 tablespoon	240
potato chips	1 ounce	250
cheese, Cheddar	1.5 ounces	275
tuna, canned	3 ounces	285–500
olives, black	2 ounces	385
ham, cured	2 ounces	400–800
cheese, cottage	½ cup	400
pancakes, prepared	3	400–800
soy sauce	1 tablespoon	420
cheese, parmesan	1 ounce	450
frankfurter	1	450
roll, crescent, prepared	2 ounces	500
tomato juice, canned	6 ounces	500
pizza	1 slice	500–1,000
cheese, American	1.5 ounces	650
pickle, dill	2 ounces	700
hamburger, prepared (Big Mac, Whopper)	1	1,000
spaghetti and meatballs, canned	7.5 ounces	1,000
soup, canned, prepared	10 ounces	1,000–1,500
TV dinner	11 ounces	1,000–2,000

Sodium Labeling

Beginning on July 1, 1986, the FDA will require food manufacturers to list the milligrams of sodium per serving on all nutrition labels. Words such as "low sodium" on a label have not always meant a great deal, but as of that date the FDA will require the standard terminology listed below. Note that "unsalted" does not mean sodium-free.

Claim on Label	FDA Requirement
Low sodium	Less than 140 mg per serving
Very low sodium	Less than 35 mg per serving
Sodium free	Less than 5 mg per serving
Reduced sodium	75% or greater reduction
Unsalted	No salt added

Source: University of California, Berkeley Wellness Letter, Volume 2, No. 7, April, 1986. Health Letter Associates, P.O. Box 412, NY, NY 10012

or tasteless. But if you are faithful to your experiment, you will discover that your taste buds will adjust so well that in a few weeks you will not miss the salt. Rather, your taste buds may be suspicious or even offended by the amount your tongue once demanded. And you will not comfortably tolerate so much again—unless and until you fall back into your old habits.

Seasonings and Spices

For some reason few diet and nutrition books say much about potential damage from condiments and irritating seasonings in the American diet. Nor do we intend to belabor them here. We distinguish between them and healthful herbs mentioned later in this chapter. But it should be caution enough to most of us to learn that most spices irritate the stomach and in time damage its lining. *To the extent that they cause damage,* they also interfere with your normal digestion and your best disposition. They saddle you with increased irritability and nervousness.

In experiments on rats, Drs. Bernell and Marjorie Baldwin found that certain irritating spices cause abnormal heart activity, increased blood pressure, and eventually retching and vomiting. They concluded that "some common spices can have significant detrimental effects on nerve, brain, heart, blood pressure, and stomach."[2] In a series of animal experiments the Drs. Baldwin found that mustard, cloves, cinnamon, and black pepper all created stomach lesions, with black pepper responsible for the largest—over four times as large as those created by mustard and much larger than the sores from cloves and cinnamon. Irritability, loss of weight, and slowing of brain activity were among other reported results.[3]

They also reported on several other studies which support their findings: "Cloves, cinnamon, and allspice contain eugenol, or oil of cloves."[4] "Eugenol damages the lining (mucosal barrier) of the stomach, making it more susceptible to ulcer formation."[5] Cinnamon contains, in addition to eugenol, oil of cinnamon, which causes inflammation and corrosion of the lining of the stomach and upper intestines.[6]

"Black pepper contains piperidine, a chemical normally used in making rubber and fuels, but which in the body causes increased release of a body hormone that stimulates the stomach to make more hydrochloric acid."[7] Mustard oil is "an active irritant of the stomach lining."[8]

You will be pleasantly surprised how the taste buds can be soothed or even slightly fooled by the clever use of herbs, either fresh or dried, which are not irritating—a list almost twice as long as the list of harmful condiments. See Recipe section in back of book which includes combinations of some of these herbs which substitute very well for the tastes we have come to enjoy.

This is another illustration of the principle that a re-education of our tastes will not only keep our bodies in better shape to the glory of God but also help us to better appreciate and prepare for our heavenly diet of wholesome, natural foods—fruits, grains, nuts, and vegetables—prepared in as wholesome a way as possible.

Supplements

A relative, very dear to us, has been working on us for years to take a lot of vitamin supplements. First he lauds one brand, then another. He has a great heritage of sound health, and admits he has squandered some of it. Yet he still finds it easier to take vitamin supplements in various forms than he does to arrange a sound diet. Is it likely that his supplemental intake stands in well for the vitamins and minerals directly from wholesome food? The answer is *no*. Scientists pretty well agree that there is no substitute for a well-balanced diet. And high quality, nutritious food is a great deal cheaper in the long run, than vitamins or doctor bills. See chart on page 82 which lists the kinds of foods that supply these vital nutrients to the body.

What *is* likely is that taking any nutrient *supplement* will imbalance other nutrients. Phosphorous and sodium depress calcium levels in the blood as does protein. Zinc in high doses depresses copper and can lead to anemia, for copper is required in making red blood cells. Excess protein makes one need more Vitamin B-12 and Vitamin A. Overdosing with vitamins C and E can suppress Vitamin A. Vitamin C in prolonged overdose can also suppress calcium absorption. And sugar uses up several B vitamins.

Psychiatrist Andrew H. Mebane recently reported that amino acid supplements can stimulate your brain or thought processes in unfortunate ways.[9] He cited one patient who was taking up to four grams of the amino acid L'glutamine daily for three weeks. He developed grandiose illusions, total insomnia, and uncontrolled sex drive. He became psychotic. Yet his hallucinations and complaints

CHART OF NUTRIENTS

RIBOFLAVIN

Food	Amount	mg.
Turnip greens	1 c.	0.60
Collards	1 c.	0.48
Milk	1 c.	0.48
Mustard greens	1 c.	0.27
Figs	10	0.25
Kale	1 c.	0.24
Dandelions	1 c.	0.22
Soybeans	1 c.	0.18
Lentils	1 c.	0.12
Rutabagas	1 c.	0.12
Almonds	12	0.10
Baked beans	1 c.	0.08
Blackstrap	1 T.	0.05

THIAMINE

Food	Amount	mg.
Grains		
Rye, whole, cooked	¾ c.	0.47
Wheat germ	1 T.	0.2–0.4
Rice, brown, cooked	½ c.	0.29
Sweet corn	½ c.	0.20
Whole wheat, cooked	¼ c.	0.15–0.198
Rolled oats, cooked	⅔ c.	0.104–0.231
Whole wheat bread	1 slice	0.072–0.12
Legumes		
Split peas	½ c.	0.87
Soybeans, dried, cooked	½ c.	0.36
Soy flour	½ c.	0.3–0.6
Peas, fresh	½ c.	0.27–0.495
Lima beans, cooked	½ c.	0.25–0.35

IRON
(Note that milk is a poor source of iron.)

Food	Amount	mg
Mustard greens, cooked	⅓ c.	5.6
Turnip greens, cooked	⅓ c.	3.5
Navy beans, cooked	½ c.	3.1
Swiss chard, cooked	½ c.	3.1
Lentils, cooked	½ c.	2.9
Soybeans, cooked	½ c.	2.5
Apricots, dried	4–6 halves	2.3
Loganberries, fresh	½–¾ c.	2.1
Molasses	1 T.	1.9
Prunes, dried	4–5	1.8
Peaches, dried	2 halves	1.8
Egg	1	1.6
Sweet potato, baked	1 large	1.4
Avocado	½ medium	1.4
White potato	1 small	1.1
Bread, whole wheat	1 slice	0.9
Milk, whole	1 c.	0.2

Food	Amount	mg
Fruits		
Avocado	½ medium	0.1–0.2
Prunes	4–5 medium	0.088–0.113
Nuts		
Brazil nuts	2 medium	0.158
Greens		
Collards	½ c.	0.22
Turnip greens	½ c.	0.138–0.18
Miscellaneous		
Brewer's yeast	1 T.	0.5–0.8
Milk	1 c.	0.096–0.156

Source: *Eat for Strength*, Uchee Pines Institute, Rt. 1, Box 273, Seale, AL 36875.

FOOD SOURCES OF THE VITAMINS

Vitamins	Sources
A	Green and yellow vegetables and fruits.
B_1	(Thiamine) Whole grains, legumes, nuts, greens.
B_2	(Riboflavin) Greens, wheat, vegetables.
B_3	(Niacin) Whole grains, nuts.
B_6	(Pyridoxin) Wheat, nuts, legumes, cabbage, bananas
	(Pantothenic acid) Legumes, wheat.
	(Biotin) Legumes, mushrooms.
	(Folic acid) Green vegetables, wheat.
	(Choline) Whole grains.
C	Greens, peppers, citrus fruits, cabbage, tomatoes, potatoes.
D	Sunshine: A fair-skinned person needs only a 6″ square of skin exposed daily to the sun for 1 hour. The darker the skin the longer the exposure needed.
E	Vegetable oils, whole grains, vegetables.
K	Cabbage, cauliflower, spinach.

Source: *Eat for Strength*, Uchee Pines Institute, Rt. 1, Box 273, Seale, AL 36875.

disappeared within a week after stopping these supplements. Another man had become hyperactive and sleepless until he ended his L'glutamine spree. This is not to say that amino acids should never be taken, but that they can alter brain function. They should be taken only under a physician's care.

Some physicians apparently dote on Vitamin B-12 shots to "give their patients energy." The University of California, Berkeley, *Wellness Letter* strongly urges that you look again if you are in such a program. Although even massive doses are unlikely to harm you, they may do considerable damage to your pocketbook.[10] You need no more than one tenth of a microgram daily. If you are a total vegetarian (vegan) and have need for B-12, Weimar's Dr. Crane suggests that you do as many orientals do: Eat some sea weed, or such fermented soy products as *miso* or *wakame;* or yet simply buy a jar of B-12 tablets at a per-day cost of "less than a penny." In any event we now know that microflora in the small intestine produce all of the vitamin B-12 most of us need.[11]

Does that mean that we should not take any supplements at all? We suggest that you counsel with an experienced physician who best understands your needs. Probably no pharmacologist or biochemist living is capable of assessing fully one's needs in the absence of signs of frank vitamin deficiency or toxicity. There is considerable reason to suggest that vitamin and mineral supplements should be treated as medicines, to be prescribed by physicians who thoroughly understand their use and potentials.

Carefully controlled dosages of vitamins and other supplements may be justified after long neglect or serious illness has depleted your body stores. Yet the best scientific advice we have found strongly suggests that eating good foods—containing your needed nutrients—is far better and less expensive in money and health than the continued use of vitamins.

Vitamins: Is More Better?

Many vitamin "addicts" assume that if a little is good, a lot must be better. But megadoses of vitamins can actually poison you! To ingest these supplements without professional advice is to take a risk, sometimes a serious one. Dr. William Patterson of the University of Missouri Health Sciences Center describes a middle-aged man who was so anemic that he was diagnosed as having "preleukemia." As he was about to undergo chemotherapy for this "cancer," another specialist found that he had been taking massive doses of zinc for prostate trouble. Within two months after he stopped the zinc supplements, and without chemotherapy, his blood tests became normal. Some believe that the overdosing of zinc prevented normal absorption of copper—the very element his body required for overcoming his anemia.

Physicians at New York City's Coney Island Hospital warn that many are overdosing on vitamins, some of them on physicians' orders. Because an older woman had broken a bone, she was being given 150,000 international units (IU's) of Vitamin D supplements daily, although the normal dosage was only 400. These dosages of D built up her blood calcium to a dangerously high level. Such hypercalcemia may result in coma. Large consumption of Vitamin A or D also can cause people to lose their hair.

One Coney Island doctor observed that some physicians are unaware that such small dosages as 400 IU are not normally available in prescription pharmacies, except in such packaging as multivitamins. This means, he says, that much larger pharmacological doses, from 25,000 to 50,000, might be given unless the physician is specific or the individual is taking vitamins without prescription.

Some years ago we talked at length with Dr. Linus Pauling, the Nobel Laureate who has become world-known for advocating large dosages of Vitamin C as well as for his advocacy of peace. Although we occasionally use C supplements, we somehow do not yet find enough evidence to support his level of enthusiasm. We prefer *whenever possible* to obtain C from citrus and similar sources. We also prefer to derive our Vitamin D from the sun and feel sorry for those who do not share enough sunlight to provide the D they need. These are reasons we suggest that you counsel with your physician, and be careful not to overdo the use of vitamin supplements.

Additives

Additives come in thousands of forms and families, but the U.S. Food and Drug Administration could find only about 150 out of 25,000 it could be sure were harmless, and all but 400 were considered dangerous.[12] We do not know of any that we can conscientiously recommend in this book for general use. There may be occasions in prepared foods where they are absolutely necessary, and where their damage may not be so great as to proscribe their use, yet in general all counsel we have received dictates: "Avoid them wherever possible."

Herbs

Herbs undoubtedly have many uses. Some are poisonous, others, helpful and even enriching in your life. Some are of course medicinal, as for example, in our family peach tree leaf tea has proven to be one of the best treatments for certain diseases or irritations of the urinary tract. But this is not a medical handbook. We suggest at least two sources for information on herbs and particularly their medicinal use: (1) *The Honest Herbal* by Dr. Varro Tyler (George F. Stickley Co., Philadelphia) and *Health Plants of the World* by Francesco Bianchin; and Francesco Corbetta (Newsweek Books, New York). See Chapter 12 for word on herbal teas.

Leavens

The most common leavening agents are yeast, baking powder, and baking soda. Yeast, a living fungus, dies when bread or rolls are baked. Its cells make the little bubbles that make bread rise. Otherwise it would sink and become very hard in the oven, much like the "bread" from which they grind the well-known "Grape Nuts."

Yeast is nutritious, but its greatest contribution is likely its releasing of minerals present in the grains. Zinc, for example, is more easily assimilated in our digestive tract if wheat is treated with yeast.

If you have been taking antibiotics, remember that they kill the bacterial flora which compete with yeast for space in your body. The result may be a takeover by yeast that often results in "yeast infection" which can result in infections of the mouth, vagina and gastrointestinal (GI) tract. One important suggestion is in order, whether or not you are on antibiotics: Let your fresh-baked bread or rolls stand for *at least* a day or two before you eat them, to insure that the yeast has thoroughly done its processing job. The lingering effects of the fresh yeast may otherwise retard digestion and harm certain of the B-vitamin content of the grain.[13] After 24 to 48 hours—preferably 48 or longer—the bread may be heated either in foil or a covered pan at about 250 degrees, and will be at least as tasty as if fresh out of the oven.

Baker's yeast, generally speaking, is the only common leaven which does not either harm nutrients in the food or leave an irritating residue in your system. For those who don't mind the disease risks inherent in eggs these days, beaten egg whites do offer an alternative to yeast.[14]

Baking powders are not in most cases considered healthful. This is particularly true of the alum-based powders and of standard baking soda. Alum-related powders, with their aluminum content, pose potential hazards for defective bone formation, dementias of Parkinson and Alzheimer types, iron loss, damage to hemoglobin in our red blood cells and possibly to the central nervous system. But the safest all-round dough-raiser appears to be yeast—even safer than non-alum powders.

10

How to Start a Change in Nutrition

A homemaker in Lansing, Michigan, told us how she had become so excited when she really studied the subject of nutrition for her family that she went home, threw out all the "harmful" things she had in her cupboard, and immediately changed her cooking style. Both her husband and her children rebelled. Though some may be able to handle this abrupt change in lifestyle, she found that it is not generally the best way to go.

The nutritionist of the family is usually the mother and it pays for her to be cautious about any change in lifestyle without the cooperation of her family. Even if her family says, "Okay," she needs to understand that her efforts may not always be enthusiastically received. Taste habits do not give up easily. Unless a serious health problem exists that needs immediate treatment, the reform in diet should be gradual, starting with removing the most harmful things and proceeding "with all deliberate speed" to a better way.

Probably the most important first step is to study the situation thoroughly with your husband on the basis of principle and together make a decision to change. You must see the reasons and really want to change. You can be assured that God who established these divine laws will cooperate and will help to strengthen your will. As far as the rest of the family is concerned, it is better to educate, educate, educate, than to legislate.

Self-Discipline

Millie Cooper, wife of Dr. Kenneth Cooper, the aerobics authority, says in her lectures, "You will never have success in your personal life, your physical life, or your emotional life unless you are disciplined." Both Ken and Millie feel that their number one priority is to allow God to lead in all aspects of their lives.

Attention to other natural laws involved in a lifestyle alteration come much more easily than a change in nutrition. The reason lies largely in our perverted tastes which have been driving our appetites, perhaps for years. This hard taskmaster will not give up without a valiant struggle against the will. Also those of us who were repeatedly lectured as children when we dawdled or stalled in eating a particular food, might have heard, "Eat it; it's good for you." This could have given us a hang-up, causing us to feel that anything wholesome couldn't possibly taste good.

How Change Comes

We can tell you by experience that in time your tastes will change so that things you once loved, you will dislike—fried foods will taste too greasy, highly salted foods too salty, white breads too soft or mushy, and sweets too icky-sweet. For example, after we stopped using certain items in our home, we didn't necessarily stop all of it when we were with family or friends or eating at restaurants (we thought that would be almost impossible), but we did the best we could and tried to choose the best available food.

As time went on, we found that more people than ever, including restaurant operators, were paying attention to good nutrition and we were able to be more selective. Now when eating out, we usually order a baked potato and go to the salad bar or just settle for the salad bar, especially in the states where spraying the fruits and vegetables with a chemical is illegal.

We know of one person who decided not to eat anything at all until he could enjoy the best food. Indeed, many of us have never allowed ourselves to get hungry or learn to control our appetite. Natural foods taste much better when you are really hungry. And you *can* change your tastes, but it takes decision, perseverance, and retraining—only about three weeks for most people.

In eliminating foods from your diet that you know are not good for you, the simplest procedure is never to buy them. If you truly study to make food attractive and tasty in a healthful way, you will relish your food and not miss the more harmful things.

Eating between Meals

"Cold Turkey" may be the only way to go here, because even the best of snacks disrupts the digestive system. Your family will relish wholesome, simple food better when the appetite has not been hampered by snacks. When you "think" you are hungry between meals, try a drink of cool tap water. Most of us do not drink half enough of this most important liquid of all. Read carefully Chapter 12, "Liquids Inside and Out," to find out why.

Caffeine and Sugar Drinks

Though possibly better than alcohol or tobacco because they harm no one but yourself, these are probably the most common and devastating habits of modern times and may be some of the most difficult to break. There are some herb teas or cereal coffees which along with water can help to alleviate the habit of tea or coffee, and fruit juices (without sweetening of any kind) can substitute for sodas and sugared drinks if needed with some meals, but even fruit juice should not be used between meals and it should be limited at meals. And we shall shortly point out that even many herb teas are harmful.

Animal Products

Cut down as you move closer to cutting out. Start eliminating red meats and fatty meats such as liver, kidney, hamburger, lunch meats, pork, and lamb. Substitute fish and chicken. Then substitute peas, lentils, a variety of beans and whole grain casseroles for main dish or protein and if you need variety use analogs (manufactured "vegetarian" meat substitutes). They are of course processed foods, but do have an advantage only of not being diseased. Dilute whole milk with nonfat milk (can be made from the powdered) or buy 2% milk and try soy or nut milks for diluting. Eventually get down to no-fat milk, if any. Feel your way on how fast you can do this, but proceed systematically. Limit each person to two eggs per week and be sure the eggs are thoroughly cooked. Choose low-fat, unprocessed cheeses, if any.

Refined Fats

This step is probably the easiest for the cook to handle, and again it is best to go easy on oils and shortenings, including even corn or safflower margarines. Buy the best quality of non- or partially hydrogenated margarine you can find for those guests or family members who "can't get along without it." In the meantime you may wean your family away from heavy use of margarine by using various spreads—sugarless fruit spreads made by blending combinations of dried fruits and water or drained unsweetened canned fruits and other spreads given in recipes. Serve low fat cottage cheese thinned and blended with skim milk and add your favorite seasoning for "sour cream" on baked potatoes. Because of disease danger and other factors, many people are also eventually eliminating dairy products.

Forego all fried foods, including the ones you sometimes buy, such as nuts roasted in oil, chips, or other processed foods. Bake, broil, or steam things you used to fry. Most everyone loves a baked potato. Try hash browns without grease by grating cooked potatoes with onions into a teflon frying pan. Instead of salt, try seasoning with onion powder. Cover and cook over medium-low heat until brown on the bottom. Then turn and cover again to brown the other side.

If you don't have Silverstone, or similar nonstick baking pans, use Pam, liquid lecithin (thinly spread with the fingers and then wiped mostly off with a paper towel) or similar product if you need to bake something which might stick such as bread, muffins or cookies. A mixture of 1 tbsp. of lecithin granules and about 2 tbsp. of water will keep in the refrigerator two or three weeks.

Try to omit oil in all recipes and especially in seasoning cooked vegetables. More often than not, your family will not know the difference.

If you use eggs, hard-cook, poach or bake them, long enough to be sure that all germs are killed—at least twenty minutes. This helps to avoid leukosis.

As much as you like to sautee your onions, try steaming them in the microwave or heavy pan with or without a small amount of water. If you start them with low heat, watch them carefully, and stir frequently, you can do it without any water.

Make gravy without oil by bringing seasoned liquid (vegetable juice, low-fat milk or water) to a boil. Be careful not to boil over or scorch the milk. Make a thin paste with a small amount of water and sufficient flour to thicken, blending either by hand or in a blender and add gradually to boiling mixture while stirring constantly. For brown gravy, flour can be dextrinized (lightly toasted) in the oven or frying pan to add flavor and color and seasoned with vegetable beef-like seasoning.

Grains

Substitute whole, instead of refined, grains as quickly as practicable. If you anticipate resistance from your family, start by substituting partial whole grain products for white and gradually increase the proportion. If you buy commercially baked bread, note that the first ingredient listed on the label is the largest. You probably will not notice the difference between whole wheat and white pasta if you cook it well.

Sugar or Honey

Unfortunately, American society has formed the bad habit of thinking a meal should end in something sweet. Until that habit can be overcome, you may need a substitute. Though fruits often satisfy the "sweet tooth," fresh fruit after a vegetable meal could create unnecessary gas and other intestinal distress for any with a weak digestion. Yet there are exceptions. Some foods commonly considered vegetables may be classified at least as accurately as fruits, as for example tomatoes.

If you can't resist making your favorite cookies or pie occasionally, *cut your sugar in half or less*. Wherever possible, use dates, raisins or other natural sweeteners instead of refined sugars. Many of our friends have found that their families either do not know the difference or actually prefer the natural way.

Cereals

Eliminate all dry cereals containing sugar. Fortunately there are a few left—possibly Grape-nuts, Shredded Wheat, and puffed grains. Try making your own granola without sugar or honey, but using raisins, date pieces, nuts, and seeds just before serving instead. Then enjoy your cereal with unsweetened applesauce, sliced bananas or other fruit on top. Also use whole-grain cereals, cooked in a double-boiler in the morning or in a crock pot overnight. Brown rice, oatmeal, mixed grain cereals (flaked, ground or cracked), and millet, cooked with little or no salt, are delicious this way.

Salt

Though some salt is acceptable, try using less. Some of our friends simply leave the salt shaker off the table. Read labels and just don't buy foods high in sodium, soda, baking powder, salt or hydrolized vegetable protein.

Budgeting

In the long run the natural food route is a real economy. You can learn to look for bargains, but always choose quality food. Wilted or partially decayed fruits or vegetables should not be used. See Chapter 3, "God's Original Diet," on how to care for foods you buy. Many towns have thrift shops where you can purchase day-old bread. We often buy a dozen loaves or so at a time, freeze some, and make much of it into zwieback through slow heat in the oven until it dries out and is very slightly browned. I like it as well as any breakfast food when Dorothy makes it from 100 percent whole wheat bread. Try until you find one you like.

Even though canned and frozen home-grown foods retain a high percentage of nutritional value for use during the winter, most of you need or want to buy some fresh things. Watch for specials when produce is in season. You don't have to buy bananas, grapes or broccoli when they are at double price. Apples and cabbage may be your alternate. And of course foods like hard-shell squashes keep very well in a cool place.

You probably already are buying generic foods, although in some stores they do not represent much of a saving. The main thing is to get full value. Some suggest it is better to use old-fashioned oats instead of the quick-fix, pre-cooked kind. Use only whole-grained breads. Don't pay for foods which have been stripped of their vitamins and minerals.

Though most healthful ingredients can be found at health food stores, they are often expensive. Such stores sometimes handle items that may be faddish rather than truly healthful and if their volume of sales is not great enough, some of their products may not be really fresh. We have found some special places which handle health foods in bulk at reasonable prices and we have also participated in a food co-op where families order in quantity at wholesale prices and then divide it. The latter is usually the cheapest but takes a little more time and leadership.

How you plan, buy, store, and use food has significant health and monetary consequences. Be aware of quality and use your imagination to make meals tasty and attractive, "gathering up the fragments" and creatively incorporating them into your meals "that nothing be wasted."

Recipes

Dorothy has books and boxes of recipes which represent our "progress." And, of course, there are far too many to print here. Yet we give you a few examples in the appendix of how she handles food—omitting oil, cutting down or alternating sweeteners and seasonings, avoiding overcooking, and otherwise preparing food, bearing in mind both our tastes and our bodies.

Healthy eating need not be boring!

11

What Goes in Must Come Out . . . Healthfully

A few years ago in central Africa, a wealthy tribal king became so constipated that his life was in danger. He traveled over the world with his royal entourage, from leading American clinics to medical centers in England and spas on the Continent. Yet for many months he had not enjoyed that special feeling of relief which follows a beautifully designed process called "peristalsis." To be deprived of this finely tuned process is common in the Western world, although not so common to Africa. Later in this chapter we will come back to the king.

It is a topic which most of us feel is too dirty or unpleasant to discuss. Let's not give in to the stupidity of ostriches and bury our heads in the sand. Your intestines are an incredibly beautiful machine that should not be abused. It is not the backyard septic tank or the city sewer system, but a strong and tender system which should not be scarred. We dare not ignore it if we want good health. *We need urgently to discuss it*—as a matter of life and death. When we do, we will find how cleansing and pleasant it can be. More later on the king.

Gracious Peristalsis

Peristalsis is that "operation digestion" inside your body's winding pipeline which carries your food along through a series of tubes, stomach, and channels with their digestive processes. If your proteins, fats, carbohydrates, vitamins, and minerals are available in the right amounts and qualities, they extract all the goodies from your food and make them into good blood. The remainder, or waste, then is ushered out by a tickling inside you that all children and adults should welcome and act on immediately, if possible.

It is one of the brighter experiences of the day for your infant in diapers. It is that wormlike movement of the intestines which forces its contents out. It is that special urge down inside for a bowel movement which you should cultivate on as regular a basis as possible. It should never be delayed unless absolutely necessary, lest there result a thickness and heaviness which not only clogs the bowel itself, but also incurs a potential strain on the rectum, inviting hemorrhoids which afflict so many of your neighbors today.

Some Colon Products

Many laymen and some physicians assume that because a stool is small, it is easier on you. Not so. If, though relatively small, it is dense, heavy, concentrated, it may be much harder on you than a larger, softer stool. Societies with high fiber diets—including a great deal of fresh fruit—tend to have large, floating stools, while Western communities more often evacuate small, sinking stools. Although this is no final indicator of your health, the larger, light-density stools usually predict a low rate of both colon and breast cancer as well as other Western degenerative diseases.

Nor is all intestinal gas necessarily bad. This is not to say that all gas-forming foods will agree with you, but most of them normally will. Yet fiber as eaten naturally in unrefined foods, and so vital to sound elimination, may increase rectal gas elimination. Trapped in the stool, gas helps to make it lighter, softer, less dense. So don't be distressed if your change in lifestyle produces some flatulence—gas formation.

Your bowel movements should be free, enjoyable experiences as you relieve yourself of unnecessary and unhealthful loads with all their potential for disease if they linger within you. Dr. Harold "Happy" Mourer, a Bellflower, California, physician, once told us that for your body and you, this relief should be among the happiest and friendliest experiences of your day. Constipation, on the other hand, leads to straining which in its various pressures causes diverticular disease, hiatal hernia, and even varicose veins and hemorrhoids. All of these problems are virtually unknown in developing countries.

If Hemorrhoids . . .

A side note: If you already have hemorrhoids or the misery that threatens—itching, soreness, strain during your bowel movements—we suggest three simple but important steps for cure: *First*, seek prompt medical counsel, but don't rush into surgery unless you are certain that it is needed. If you find you do need surgery, don't delay. I know from miserable personal experience the itching, discomfort, pain, and alarm associated with this condition. Yet, as with mine, your surgeon may have to do no more than lance the thrombosed hemorrhoid to release—in my case—a blood clot. *Second*, keep yourself very clean. Perhaps use some simple, mild salve during the period of your distress. Use cold water in your cleansing, for it tends to shrink rather than inflame your tissues. I found it helpful to use cold packs—ice, wrapped in a washcloth— to take down rectal swelling. If you recognize the symptoms early— itching, pain—you can usually avoid the need for surgery. *And third*, get your lifestyle in order, in balance, as we suggest in this book—in fiber-rich foods, exercise, rest, water, and all those really good things.

Cystitis. We must also mention here a bowel-related "plague" that few will discuss. Women suffer most. Because the female urethra is short, women often suffer a bladder infection called cystitis. This is usually caused by *e-coli,* a bacterium normally found in feces. If women are not careful, it will easily move from anus to vagina and invade the urethra and bladder. One female laboratory technician suggested that Dorothy advise mothers to teach little girls to wipe themselves from front to back after using the toilet, and otherwise be very careful to keep e-coli out of the wrong channels.

Fiber

Though others have tried in vain to help people understand the importance of fiber, Dr. Denis Burkitt, often called "the fiber man," is the one most often credited with successfully getting the information out to the public. He made his discoveries during his more than twenty years as a missionary doctor in Africa, as he studied the contrast between the diseases of the Western world and the primitive tribes.

This pioneer physician and surgeon found that breaking through Western prejudices—and vested interests—was a wearing task, yet God led him in mysterious ways to give new tools to preventive medicine. Interestingly enough, Dr. Burkitt discovered that as far back as the third century before Christ, Hippocrates, the father of modern medicine, and later the Persian physician Hakim—in the ninth century A.D.—both encouraged the use of coarse flour and bran because of their bowel-emptying virtues.

Fiber, especially cereal and fresh fruit fiber, is called the roto-rooter of the digestive tract. If you eat it in its natural form on a regular basis and drink at least six to eight glasses of water a day (although not with meals), as far as you are concerned the laxative industry can go out of business.

Dr. Burkitt strongly feels that the reasons usually given for varicose veins—heredity, or pregnancy, or standing for long periods—are not principal causes. He tells about the Masai tribesmen "who never sit down," and others who stand all day guarding their cattle, yet never develop varicose veins. The American Negro has them, but not his relatives in Africa. And Africans who have three times as many pregnancies as their American cousins do not get varicose veins.

Cancer

Yet diverticulitis, hernias, and varicose veins are hardly the threats that most of us find in cancer. Dr. Arthur Upton of the National Cancer Institute urges the use of natural dietary fiber—found in fruits, grains, nuts, and vegetables as near as practicable to their natural form—to reduce the risk of bowel cancer which, after lung cancer, is the second greatest cause of cancer death in North America and Western Europe.

Transit time in the intestines—the interval between the intake of food and elimination of the waste—makes much of the difference. A natural diet as prescribed in this book will produce a normal transit time of 35 hours. In contrast, a diet of refined food, especially when combined with snacking, may take 70 to 80 hours or in extreme cases even up to 120 hours to move through your body.

It is not hard to imagine the effect on your body of small, hard, pebbly stools moving slowly through the intestines and prolonging the contact time with the intestinal wall, with their carcinogenic (cancer-causing) chemicals produced by unfriendly bacteria in the bowel. On the other hand, says Dr. Burkitt, cellulose in the fiber of natural foods, once in the intestinal tract, absorbs water and swells, making the stools softer and larger, and moving them through the body promptly, in most cases entirely eliminating constipation.

Dr. Burkitt concludes, along with the National Research Council, that the incidence of total cancer could be reduced in the United States at least one-third by stopping smoking and another third through changes in diet. Among these substantially preventable diseases, he believes, is breast cancer. He notes that cancer of the breast is caused principally by excessive fat in the diet which causes an overproduction of the female hormone, estrogen.

Dr. Burkitt also reports that the amount of estrogen (excreted in the stool) is lowered as the size (bulk) of the stool is increased. He believes that this is one reason why vegetarians are less likely to have cancer than non-vegies. It has long been known that estrogen is cancer-linked. Similar cancers he lists are those of the endometrium (lining of the womb) in women and the prostate in men.

Fiber—Again—One of Your Best Friends

Because of the rarity of certain other diseases in the rural areas of the Third World and the prominence of these diseases in Western culture, Dr. Burkitt strongly feels that coronary heart disease, diabetes, appendicitis, obesity, and gallstones are also largely preventable, and that fiber is a key corrective measure.

Although the most likely cause of adult-onset diabetes is a chronic excess of empty calories of all kinds, lack of fiber also contributes to diabetes because it allows sudden release of glucose into the bloodstream—from consumption of refined sugar, honey or even fruit juices. This is especially true when these sweets are taken in between meals. On the other hand, fiber in its beautiful God-made natural packaging works like a sponge to keep sugar from being absorbed too fast.[1]

The common practice of adding bran, which has been isolated from its natural sources, to food that is depleted in fiber, probably will have some beneficial effects, but it is much more efficient and effective when eaten in its native undisrupted state, prepared with a minimum of sugars, spices, and oils. For example, whole brown rice protects from rapid blood glucose and insulin response more than ground brown rice.[2] And apples avoid insulin response considerably better than apple juice or even unsweetened applesauce.[3]

Fiber Sources

Processing of food has removed some of the most valuable, protective components of food as it comes from the plant. Natural fiber is one of those important constituents whose destruction has left a long train of ills among the "more advanced" population. *Meat, eggs, dairy products, and seafoods have no fiber at all.* Nor have refined oil, including margarine and mayonnaise, and refined sugar.

Fruits

The type of dietary fiber of course varies in different foods. Apples and most fruits contain *pectin,* the well-known ingredient in fruit used in jelly-making, but also valuable in the diet to aid in regulating cholesterol. The apple, especially, is well accepted as a help to control both diarrhea and constipation. Remarkably, it also helps to prevent lead poisoning,[4] it reduces the absorption and deposition of radioactive strontium 90 in the body,[5] and it is an anti-bacterial agent which attacks staphylococci, streptococci, and other bacteria.[6] So eat plenty of apples with the skin on (unless you have diarrhea), and oranges with all or part of the white membrane, and an abundance of other fruits.

Each fiber has its place. That in fruit and vegetables is softer than that in grains and is broken down by enzymes in the small bowel, while cereal fiber moves on virtually unchanged into the large bowel where its value is greatest. Unrefined cereal foods have an excellent effect. For example, a loaf of whole wheat bread has from about three to eight times as much fiber as white bread, yet it has eight times the effect on the *bulkiness* of the stool.[7] Some of these cereal fibers include: Oat bran with its high *hemicellulose* content, wheat bran which is high in *cellulose,* and many other cereal fibers. The *gums* and mucilages in legumes (peas,

Dietary Fiber Content in 100 Grams of

Food	*Grams of Fiber*	*Household Unit*
Breads, Flours and Grains		
Barley, pearl, boiled	2.2	unavailable
Bran, wheat, 100%	44.0	1⅔ C
Flour, 100% wheat	9.6	⅚ C
Flour, all purpose	3.4	5/7 C
Oatmeal, raw	7.0	1¼ C
Oatmeal, cooked	0.8	5/12 C
Rice, boiled white	0.8	⅝ C
Soy flour, full fat	11.9	1⅙ C
Soy flour, low fat	14.3	1 1/7 C
Whole wheat bread	8.5	4 slices
White bread	2.7	4 slices
Cereals		
All-Bran	26.7	1¾ C
Cornflakes	11.0	4 C
Grapenuts	7.0	3½ oz.
Puffed Wheat	15.4	7 C
Rice Krispies	4.5	3½ C
Shredded Wheat	12.3	4 biscuits
Special K	5.5	5 C
Rye Crispbread	11.7	not available, but 5 triple Ry-Krisp weigh 110 gms.
Vegetables		
Asparagus, boiled	1.5	⅔ C
Beans, green, boiled	3.4	1 C
Beans, baked, canned in tomato sauce	7.3	½ C
Beans, boiled, kidney	7.4	⅖ C
Broccoli, boiled	4.1	⅔ C
Brussels Sprouts, boiled	2.9	6 to 7
Cabbage, winter, raw	3.4	1 C
Cabbage, winter, boiled	2.8	⅗ C
Carrots, boiled	3.1	⅔ C
Cauliflower, boiled	1.8	⅞ C
Celery, raw	1.8	1 C
Celery, boiled	2.2	⅘ C
Corn	4.7	⅖ C
Lentils, split, boiled	3.7	½ C
Lettuce	1.5	3½ oz.
Peas, boiled	5.2	⅔ C
Peas, split, boiled	5.1	3½ oz.
Potatoes, baked in skin, flesh only	2.5	1, 2¼–2½" diameter
Potatoes, boiled	1.0	1 medium
Spinach, boiled without added water	6.3	1¾ C
Sweet potatoes, boiled	2.3	½ potato 5" by 2"
Tomatoes, raw	1.5	1, 2⅖" diameter
Turnips, boiled	2.2	⅔ C
Turnip greens, boiled	3.9	⅔ C
Fruits		
Apples, raw, peeled	2.0	1 small
Apples, baked without sugar & skin	2.5	1 small
Apples, stewed without sugar	2.1	1 small
Apple peel	3.7	not available

SELECTED FOODS, IN HOUSEHOLD UNITS*

Food	Grams of Fiber	Household Unit
Apricots, raw, without pits	2.1	2–3 medium
Avocado	2.0	½, 3¼ by 4"
Bananas	3.4	1 small, 6"
Blackberries, raw	7.3	⅝ C
Cherries, without pits	1.7	15 large, 25 small
Cranberries, raw	4.2	1 C
Dates, without pits	8.7	10 medium
Figs, raw	2.5	2 large or 3 small
Figs, dried	18.3	5 medium or ⅔ C cut
Grapes, black, including skin	0.3	22–24 medium
Grapes, white including skin	0.9	22–24 medium
Grapefruit	0.6	½ medium, 4" in diameter
Lemons, including skin	5.2	1 small
Loganberries, raw	6.2	⅔ C
Melons, cantaloupe	1.0	¼ of melon, 5" in diameter
Melons, honeydew	0.9	¼ of melon, 5" in diameter
Olives	4.4	¾ C sliced
Oranges, without skin	2.0	1 sm. 2½" in diameter
Peaches, raw	1.4	1 medium
Peaches, dried	14.3	½ C
Pears, eating, weighted with skin and core	1.7	½ pear 3 by 2½" in diameter
Pineapple, fresh	1.2	¾ C
Pineapple, canned with syrup	0.9	1 large slice
Prunes, dried raw	16.1	8 large
Prunes, pitted, stewed without sugar	8.1	5 medium with 2 T juice
Raisins	6.8	⅝ C
Raspberries, raw	7.4	¾ C
Rhubarb, stewed, with or without sugar	2.2	⅜ C
Strawberries	2.2	10 large
Tangerines, without peel	1.9	1 large or 2 small

NUTS

Almonds, without shell	14.3	⅔ C
Brazil nuts, without shell	9.0	⅓ C
Chestnuts, without shell	6.8	½ C scant
Coconut, fresh	13.6	1 C
Coconut, dried	23.5	1⅔ C
Peanuts, fresh, without shell	8.1	not available
Peanut butter	7.6	6–7 T
Walnuts, without shell	5.2	1 C halves

EGGS	0	
FATS	0	
MEATS	0	
MILK	0	

* Dietary fiber values of 100 gram portions are taken from Paul, A. A. and D. A. T. Southgate, *McCance and Widdowson's The Composition of Foods,* Fourth revised and extended ed. Her Majesty's Stationery office, London, 1978.

Conversions of household measures of 100 gram portions are from Pennington, J. A. T. and H. N. Church, *Bowes and Church's Food Values of Portions Commonly Used,* 13th ed. J. B. Lippincott Co., Phila. 1980, and Adams, C. F. *Nutritive Value of American Foods in Common Units.* Agriculture Handbook No. 456, U.S.D.A., Washington, D.C., 1975.

beans, lentils, and so on) additionally help reduce intestinal bacteria, serum cholesterol levels of the blood, and transit time through the bowel.

Though you will not need to keep track of how much fiber you eat if you stay away from refined foods, you might like to know that Dr. Burkitt recommends that we eat 40 grams of dietary fiber each day. We include the chart on pages 100 and 101 to help you see how you are doing.

Balance in Your Meals

A well-balanced diet of fresh, natural, fiber-filled foods, lightly cooked and seasoned, as we note in Chapter 3, "God's Original Diet," then is important to healthy bowels and efficient elimination. We deliberately refer to this need many times, from different angles in this book. If you take this as seriously as we hope, you will have a much healthier life and fewer days in the hospital.

This not only makes clinical common sense, but it is well supported by top scientific groups. And those who lead in the great American empty-calorie-junk-food marathon scarcely try to defend the indefensible. The National Research Council of the National Academy of Science advises us all to eat more fresh fruits, vegetables, and whole-grain cereal products daily if we want to avoid colon cancer.

This does not mean that we should overeat, but rather choose wisely what we *do* eat—and when. For example, go easy on fried foods and fatty diets, refined and salty items and those condiments and sauces which irritate your digestive tract. Unpeeled apples, baked potatoes eaten in their skins with little or no grease, whole grains with their natural bran, very little refined fat—dairy butter, oils (especially hydrogenated or high temperatured), margarine, mayonnaise—make for easy, healthy relief. Become more friendly with the cabbage family—broccoli, Brussels sprouts, cabbage, cauliflower—and its "trigger molecules" that help turn cancers away through their *indoles* which increase the production of enzymes thus helping to inactivate cancer-producing substances. Yellow and green vegetables in general, fresh or not overcooked, are also vitamin-filled guerrillas against cancer.

Some Exceptions

Although such a dietary direction should be the rule, sometimes emergencies demand exceptions. For example, while apples are usually much more healthful when eaten unpeeled, you may better eat your apples peeled if you have diarrhea, because of the natural laxative effect of fresh apple peels. I remember well an occasion while traveling near the Arctic Circle in the northern reaches of Norway when I desperately reached for a drink that I normally would never imbibe. I was simultaneously taken with diarrhea and vomiting. The airline stewardess had a chalklike medicine for the nausea, but as an emergency therapy for diarrhea I drank a can of Coca Cola, which had an almost immediate effect of stopping me up. This has happened to me several times in traveling over the world, possibly because of a constipating (or paralyzing) effect of the sugar and caffeine.

But one of the greatest natural cathartics or elimination aids is *water,* especially warm water, drunk between meals—not less than thirty minutes before eating nor within an hour afterward, unless you don't mind diluting your gastric juices which are needed to digest your meals. A pint to a quart of lukewarm water drunk a half hour or more before breakfast almost always works as a natural laxative, usually cleansing the system within the hour.

You often hear one say, "But I drink a lot of juice." In the first place, juice does not substitute for water in the body any more than it does for washing your dishes in the sink. In fact, fresh fruit eaten whole will serve you better as an internal cleanser, and it provides more balanced nutrition and natural fiber. You will find much more on this in Chapter 12, "Liquids Inside and Out."

The Troubled King

Medical authorities prescribed none of the above for the African king introduced at the beginning of this chapter. They largely prescribed cathartics and other medicines. At first they did suggest coarse bran-type foods, but his digestive tract had by now become so fragile that many common laxative foods irritated his system. There remained perhaps the best treatment of all, one so common that many physicians forget about it even if they know. It would even help strengthen his weakened and irritated organs.

One day one of the king's servants, a Christian, asked him if he would consider visiting an American physician at a mission station operated by a Protestant church on a compound a few villages distant—a place best known for its care of the native poor. The king's desperation for relief finally overcame his pride, and one day he rolled up to the mission clinic in his Rolls Royce limousine, followed by his retinue with their arms full of medical records.

The excitement at the clinic did not easily abate, for all knew of this wealthy monarch and were aware that in his preoccupation with his native religions he had not been particularly friendly to the mission. The physician nevertheless made the king as comfortable as he could and settled into his diagnosis. After detailing the long story of his world-wide quest for relief, the king sighed with an air of utter futility.

"I am here as a last desperate resort," he told the doctor.

The physician begged the king's indulgence while he looked carefully over the medical records handed him by the monarch's secretary. Then he asked, "How much water do you drink daily?"

The king looked at him with furrowed eyes. "What is this you ask?"

"I ask how much water do you drink each day?"

"Very little," answered the great one proudly. "In fact almost none at all." The secretary explained to the doctor that "The king has other things to drink." The physician knew this all too well. The water in the area was not generally good tasting or pure, and most local Africans turned from it.

Cautiously he asked the king, "Would you be offended if I prescribed a very simple remedy?"

"No," the king answered, shaking his head, but plainly showing his puzzlement.

"It is a *very* simple idea, and I will not charge you for it," assured the doctor, "but I feel sure it will help you."

"Please?" asked the king, unaccustomed to waiting for answers.

"I would like to have you drink at least six glasses of water each day, beginning today, and within a few days step up to at least eight glasses daily. Boil your water thoroughly to be sure that it is pure. And I'd like to have you for the next several weeks eat only fresh fruit, whole grains, and vegetables moderately cooked with very little oil. My wife will be glad to help your cook, if that is necessary."

Disappointed King

The king looked at him in astonishment. He had expected an exotic remedy.

"In the morning," continued the physician without hesitation, "I want you to drink from two to four glasses of warm (neither too hot or too cold) water at least a half hour before breakfast. Get to four as soon as you can. And drink either a half hour before meals or at least an hour after meals, so as not to dilute your digestive juices."

The monarch's mouth dropped. "Only water? Is that all?"

"Yes," was the answer. "That is all for now, along with the simple foods I suggested." And the doctor walked his majesty to his limousine, adding, "Please let me know in a few days how you are feeling."

Enthusiastic King

Six weeks later the king again rolled up to the clinic office. He literally bounced out of his Rolls Royce, followed by ladies and men in waiting from other vehicles, their arms now filled with gifts for the doctor and his staff.

"I apologize for the delay," the grateful ruler said with apparent embarrassment, now bowing slightly to the physician. "There have been some appointments out of the country."

Beckoning his servants to deliver the many gifts, he exclaimed, "So simple! How wonderful!" And explained that he was "cured in almost a day." But it had taken him a little longer to believe it.

The water cure fit for a king may not always be so welcome. Some prefer juices or Perrier or Coke and a doughnut or sweet roll. But like the African king—or Naaman the leper who also had a water cure—the simpler and humbler way is the least expensive and best.[8]

If you value your health and want to avoid future pain and expense, you will become much more alert to your body's need for cleansing. Your bladder and bowels will take on new meaning. For example, if you combine warm water with walking or running, be sure to keep in mind the possibility that peristalsis may arrange one of its friendly visits at an unfriendly time. So don't walk or run too far from a restroom until your bladder and bowels are relieved.

Some ask about drugstore laxatives. We answer that they may be good in their place, depending on the condition of your system and the counsel of your physician. But for the most part they are crutches and should not be used habitually unless it is impossible for you to take the proper preventive measures we have described here and in Chapter 3 (Diet).

If we do not provide sound enough conclusions and evidence, please demand the same of us. Avoid drugs as much as possible, especially those which you find have a constipating effect on you. Ask God to help reduce your stress, and to give you the strength to conquer appetite so that you are eating and drinking to *His* glory. Remember the diet of the King, *your king!*

12

Liquids Inside and Out

Trisha, an attractive, trimly dressed young California mother came to us after one of our lectures at Stanford. She was the well-educated wife of a Silicon Valley engineer who was a leader in one of the computer industries there. Her four-year-old son had serious constipation problems and almost constantly had a hacking cough.

We inquired if she had consulted a pediatrician or family physician. She had. We asked her if she kept his arms and legs warm. Yes. Did he wear something on his head when it was cold? Yes. We quizzed her about his diet, and found it to be better than average. And he was getting plenty of exercise. Then we asked how much water he drank.

"Virtually none," she replied somewhat sheepishly. "My doctor asked the same question."

"And what did you tell him?"

"He hates water!" Then, looking straight at us, she added "And I do, too!"

"That may be your problem."

"How do you mean?"

"He must have plenty of water," we pointed out, "in order to have a healthy body. And he will likely do as you do."

"But I give him lots of juices—fruit juices, vegetable juices and. . . ."

"And?"

"An occasional soft drink."

"Like what?"

"He likes Pepsi and Mountain Dew. And I do give him a lot of milk." We could see those angel wings sprouting all over her with the last sentence.

"Is his coughing productive? Is there some sputum, does he cough up mucus?"

"O yes, a lot. I guess that's what bothers me most. And he gets all stopped up at night. Bill and I have not had a good night's rest in months."

"And what do you drink?"

"Coffee, mostly, some fruit juices and an occasional Pepsi."

"And how is your own health?" we wondered out loud, looking at her pale, but otherwise beautiful complexion.

"The doctor says I'm a bit anemic, but he has prescribed some iron extract and pills, and I think I'm doing better."

Ignorant or Uninformed

For all her education and sophistication Trisha had either not known or ignored some of the most basic principles in good health . . . and child psychology. She is not at all unique. *First,* she had not learned *what* to drink, *when* to drink or *why* to drink. There would be fewer and smaller hospitals, healthier and happier people and much lower medical costs if Americans became informed, used enough common sense to realize that what goes into their bodies largely dictates what their bodies will become. The first four letters of *health* are *heal,* and both our food and drink should heal, not hurt. The Apostle Paul said they should be "to the glory of God."[1] And, *second,* she had overlooked the power of parental example.

We asked a few more questions of Trisha and answered her questions, put her in closer touch with her family doctor and sent her home. A few weeks later we received one of those special letters that shines out among the thousands which come to us every month. With her strong distaste for water, we had to be careful how to approach her. Her physician had tried and apparently failed to impress on her the urgent need for body cleansing inside as well as outside. And highly educated people are often the least teachable, so I had told her this story as a means of giving her specific advice:

The Japan Cure

A few years after World War II we found ourselves in Japan overwhelmed with the task of helping to rehabilitate Christian education in that nation. Dorothy was teaching in college and was campus hostess in addition to her preferred profession as homemaker. I was president of a Christian college which had been deeply troubled, in addition to building a church school system, and I shared in a small way in the development of the new International Christian University.

Before long I found myself coughing in the night and almost continuously spitting up mucus during the day. This went on until someone suggested that I might have tuberculosis, a dreaded disease then rampant in Japan. Scared, I headed for the Tokyo Sanitarium and Hospital, then noted for the finest of American medical care. Dr. Erwin Syphers looked me over carefully and then leveled with me.

"You are on the way to bronchiectasis," he said with a worried glance that was ominous in itself. Noting my quizzical look, he quickly explained, "You are developing a permanent infection of your bronchial tubes which could be worse than tuberculosis."

"Then what . . . ?" I reacted much like I always imagined a person newly informed that he had a fatal disease.

"I want you to do two things."

"Yes?" I expected some bitter pills and possibly an order home to America.

"I want you to drink a quart of lukewarm water every morning a half hour or more before breakfast," he admonished, "and I want to be sure you keep your extremities always warm."

I sighed with relief, but was curious about the remedies. He quickly anticipated my curiosity. "The water will literally wash you out, get rid of the unnecessary bulk and filth which accumulates in any body." We will discuss his answers about body warmth in Chapter 18, "Temperance, Stress and Trust in God."

Drinking with Meals

Within six weeks I was completely free of coughing and spitting. And now for over thirty years Dr. Sypher's simple cure has been a key factor in keeping our family from colds, influenza and chest problems. He further admonished me not to drink water or a large amount of any liquids with my meals, particularly water.

"Common sense," he counseled, "will tell you that it will dilute your gastric juices, and that is going to slow your digestion. So drink your water at least thirty minutes before eating and not until at least an hour after each meal." And he counseled that for best health and least risk of disease, I should not drink *anything* very cold or very hot. Very cold liquids interfere with the body temperatures and the normal digestive needs. Very hot drinks often cause serious damage to the throat. One of Japan's leading surgeons told me that the drinking of very hot tea was the principal reason for Japan's high incidence of throat cancer—which is many times higher than that of Americans.

We also took a few minutes to tell Trisha of Dorothy's conversion to the regular early morning and between-meal waterings. Soon all four members of our family had our jars of warm water, appropriate to our size, lined up on the drainboard each morning. And we added these items which the Tokyo story did not fully cover:

Those Un-Waters

Juices do not bring the uninhibited cleansing action which water provides. They must themselves be digested, while water can wash right on through the system, cleaning as it goes. We talk more in the chapters on diet about how fresh fruits are better cleansers than juices, and more nutritional. Yet we readily agree that fruit juices are to be desired when compared with soft drinks, coffee, tea, and for many, even milk.

Soft drinks should never enter the mouth of a child, and preferably not even an adult, unless there is an emergent need for liquids, or unless you are in a situation where that is the better part of valor or yet, unless as we point out in Chapter 11, "What Goes In Must Come Out . . . Healthfully," you are using something like Coke® as an effective constipating agent to stop diarrhea. Such drinks, like snacks, are especially harmful between meals, as also noted in our chapters on diet and regularity. More on them in the next few pages.

Milk, we repeat, a drink which most of us in the Western World have thrived on from infancy, is now coming more and more into question for several reasons. Among them, it has been found to be a carrier of disease from cows. Raw milk, particularly, has been proven to be dangerous until after sterilization, because of danger of *salmonella dublins,* a virulent strain of bacteria, dangerous to infants, the elderly and infirm.[2] Goat's milk has been less of a problem, according to some experts, because of its unique properties. We cannot verify this, for this milk has not received the attention of standard dairy products and its production has apparently been relatively too small to justify it.

Cows' milk definitely stimulates the creation of mucus (phlegm) in many, if not most, children and adults, with congestion in the nasal passages and upper respiratory area. Some physicians are now saying that milk was intended only for the early months of life—before animals and children can take a full diet of other foods. We do not suggest that it is a poison or in the class with soft drinks, but we do counsel common sense if you or your children are troubled with nasal or bronchial congestion.

Coffee and Tea

In view of her anemia, we also passed on to Trisha some recent information on coffee and tea. "Researchers have known for some time that tea can reduce iron absorption by as much as 87% when it is drunk with a meal, thereby making less iron available for body functions. Now coffee has been shown to interfere with the body's use of iron."[3] However the culprit in this iron absorption escapade is probably not caffeine, but tannic acid, a polyphenol chemical which probably causes the problem in both tea and coffee.[4]

Tufts editors also allude to *American Journal of Clinical Nutrition* report that a cup of regular drip coffee reduced iron absorption by 39 percent when drunk with a hamburger meal. This is worthy of particular note for women during their menstrual years. It appears to make no difference whether the coffee is decaffeinated or not. If you are a woman and must have your coffee, it will help a little if you eat fresh fruit or even have a glass of orange juice to reduce coffee's effect on iron absorption.

Caffeine's Other Gifts

Apart from its awakening, pick-up, stimulating effect on the central nervous system, caffeine offers a few less obvious inducements—or warnings: It can increase the heartbeat or make it irregular, increase urine production, substantially increase cholesterol level regardless of sex and whether or not you use cream, increase likelihood of birth defects and mutations, and open some blood vessels at the same time it is constricting others.[5]

Whether it is decaffeinated or not, coffee will increase your stomach's acid output. So if you have ulcers in your digestive system, your physician will insist on no coffee of any kind. These are in addition to the commonly known symptoms such as insomnia, headaches, diarrhea, nervousness, trembling, and irritability.[6]

In the March 19, 1986 issue of *The Wall Street Journal* [p. 29], John Valentine wrote that "The U.S. coffee industry has a bad case of the baby-boom blues." While consumption of gourmet coffees has increased, the overall percentage of people drinking coffee has declined 41 percent since 1962. During the same period, soft drinks showed more than 100 percent gain, moving from about 30 percent of the population to more than 60 percent, while coffee has declined to about 55 percent.

But it isn't because of the new generation's enlightenment, but rather their preferences for soft drinks—which, if anything, may be even worse because of their high sugar content in addition to the caffeine level in many of them. Some of course will debate this, considering coffee's many volatile oils and other problems besides caffeine.

Whether you take your caffeine from the cola nut or from the coffee bean, this stimulant is an enemy that not only deprives you of iron, but it is also a con artist, a salesman bent on selling you something you don't really want. It markets heart disease, cancer (possibly of the pancreas), fibrocystic breast disease and birth defects. The International Coffee Organization, like the Tobacco Institute and its anger over today's war on tobacco, claims that the research is not conclusive. Nevertheless, we pass this on as a caution in a nation which yearly turns some 2.5 billion pounds of coffee into a favorite drink.[7]

Nor does caffeine come only in the coffee cup! You will find it in diet pills, allergy pills, headache medicines, baked goods, frozen desserts, puddings, cold remedies, some teas, chocolate, and some soft drinks, especially colas. But only about 5 percent of the caffeine in colas, Dr. Pepper, and so on, comes from the cola bean. *Most of it is a gift to you as a leftover: much of the caffeine taken in the decaffeinating process goes into colas.* The baby-boom blues about coffee only means big gains for its invidious and dangerous sword, caffeine. Note also the caution on caffeine during pregnancy in Chapter 20, "When Families Are Pregnant."

Any of these drugs, such as caffeine, which stimulate the central nervous system, should be used cautiously, if at all. It is better to stay away from these stimulants which ultimately depress. For you are only robbing your body of vitality and long-term welfare of your brain.

Herbal Teas

Although the Moore family members have for most of their lives used little tea and coffee, we have freely imbibed herbal teas when our host or hostess offered them. Now we, too, have some rethinking to do if we are to believe James N. Roitman of the U.S. Department of Agriculture's Western Regional Research Center. *Comfrey* may be one of the worst, even though it is recommended by herbal authors to be therapeutic in more than 40 ailments.[8]

Dr. Roitman observes that comfrey, prepared as tea, contains dangerous levels of pyrrolizidine alkaloids which cause liver damage. He is not crying "Fire" about an occasional cup of tea, yet is warning that its use along with other teas may have a cumulative effect. The Food and Drug Administration is currently studying herbal teas for their possible toxic effects.

The University of California *Wellness Letter* recently reported that while most packaged herb teas appear to be harmless, certain of their ingredients may bring "adverse reactions" to some.[9] Most of these teas have been tested neither for safety nor healing qualities when consumed in large amounts. And now researchers are finding that some of them may contain substances as dangerous as coffee and regular tea, or more so. For example: *Chamomile* brings allergic reactions to those sensitive to ragweed or goldenrod; *sassafras* is a known carcinogen, and *nutmeg* can be toxic when brewed in large quantities. So the Wellness Letter advises consumers to drink such teas "in reasonable amounts," not as medical panaceas.

Dr. Varro Tyler, Dean of Purdue University's School of Pharmacy and Pharmaceutical Sciences warns that some teas should be avoided altogether:[10] *Lobelia*—depresses breathing, increases heartbeat, can induce coma or even death. *Wormwood*—has caused convulsions. *Sassafras*—one of its chemicals causes cancer in animals. *Comfrey*—causes cancer in animals. *Coltsfoot, mistletoe,* and *pennyroyal* are also dangerous.

Also, go easy on *senna* lest it induce diarrhea. *Raspberry* leaves have high levels of tannin which may upset your stomach, especially during pregnancy. It may even be cancer-inducing. *Chamomile* isn't as helpful as thought for upset stomachs and may be bad for those who are allergic to ragweed, asters, chrysanthemum, goldenrod and yarrow. It may be found in such products as Celestial Seasoning's Sleepy Time.

Peppermint leaf tea is often a help for indigestion, but not for small children who might feel choked. *Valerian root* may be a safer tranquilizer than synthetic drugs. But most medicinal teas are "very dilute sources of drugs." It pays to check with your physician.

We write this with a caution not to panic, but to examine carefully what you put in your body. There is almost certainly a number of uses of herbs, both outside and in, which stamp them among our most friendly health aids.

Chocolate or Cocoa

The data and biases on hot or cold chocolate range from one extreme to the other. As a food, cocoa can be damaging or not so harmful depending on the source of the cocoa bean. The caffeine content in some beans is so small as to be negligible. For example, there was found to be .329 percent of caffeine in chocolate from New Guinea, while there was only .064 percent in chocolate from Fernando Po in Africa. And theobromine varies from 1.73 percent in Nigeria down to 0.818 percent in New Guinea.[11] Although there are those ever-present caffeine and theobromine alkaloids, the main harm, some nutritionists contend, is that cocoa almost always requires substantial use of sugar, depending of course on the concentration of cocoa.

The same applies to carob, according to most candy makers we have contacted. On the other hand, some insist that carob is naturally sweeter than cocoa, and is amenable to natural sweeteners. So, while we make no pronouncements on these products, it would be best to go lightly on them if we value our health. Depending on your taste discrimination, carob may or may not take the place of chocolate in your recipes. And while we hesitate to step on the toes of our caffeine-drinking friends, there is not a single way it directly aids your health, but rather it serves a similar purpose as tobacco or alcohol or other drugs in giving a false lift.

In any event keep chocolate products away from your pets, especially dogs, for theobromine is said to be deadly for dogs, according to the Humane Society. Theobromine poisoning in dogs may bring incontinence, nervousness, and even seizures. Call your veterinarian if you observe these symptoms.

Trisha admitted that her prejudices, that is, her appetite and taste buds, had come between her and reality. She quickly saw that her example had been teaching her son and vowed that "for his sake even more than mine" she would make a new start.

"Maybe not a quart at a time," she grinned with a total change in attitude, "but we're going all the way this time."

For some of you, bottled water—or rain water if available—may be the best way to begin, considering the quality of water in many areas today. Some mothers feel forced to boil water to avoid disease or to flavor it with lemon juice because of the obnoxious taste in some areas. You will be wise to do whatever is necessary to make the water healthful and potable, but don't neglect using it both outside and in, and in adequate amounts, depending on the size of your body. You would not try washing your dishes with a single cup of water or a glass of orange juice or a soft drink. Your body is much more complex and needs a thorough flushing every day.

Many of our friends, like Trisha, tell us that they hate water. They don't, really. They like to swim in it, bathe with it, use it for their laundry. But they ignore it for the most important use of all. It has been our experience that few parents teach their children that water is their best drink. Yet it is not too late to learn.

Take It Easy

But don't overdo! We have friends who each drink a gallon of water on a normal day and more in very hot weather. And all of us should be drinking at least six to eight glasses (1–½ to 2 quarts) daily. But you may need a few days to get to your goal. Just be sure your goal is realistic.

Dr. Vernon Foster tells of a patient who was despairing because she couldn't manage more than 24 glasses of water a day.

"Twenty-four?" asked the astonished physician.

"Yes," she answered apologetically, as anxious to please her physician as she was for her own welfare, "but I don't think I can ever make 68. . . ."

Dr. Foster was at first puzzled, and then he laughed: He explained to the puzzled patient, "I said 'six to eight,' not 68."

Suddenly the idea became reasonable to her again.

J. W. McFarland, M.D., principal author of the famed "5-Day Plan to Stop Smoking," tells why water is so important to your health:[12] Your skin receives about a third of all your blood, helps regulate your body heat with its 2,000,000 sweat glands, and loses from a quart to three quarts of body fluids each day, depending upon the weather. This fluid must be replaced. You must choose whether you will do it with coffee or tea or soft drinks or . . . water. And water is what your body craves most. Your good health and mental alertness demand it. Even your body's endurance depends on it.[13]

Of course, the more water *in,* the more water *out.* You must plan for that. Some of our readers and listeners and friends tell us, "But my schedule will not permit it." Then perhaps you should change your schedule before your schedule changes you! Why not be a bit more frank with your associates, if this is your problem? We have done this and have found that some of our associates have followed our lead.

Babies, Too

Babies should be offered water between feedings from birth. They may not need it badly if breast fed, but should learn to like it and continue to drink water consistently including the early morning cleanser. It is better to change diapers oftener than to have to deal with unnecessary infections. Water is especially important to the young—who have not yet fully developed their immunities. Give your tiny tots sipping cups which do not easily spill. Get them in the habit of drinking water instead of demanding food between their regular meals. You will find more on this in our book *Home Grown Kids*.

Water Outside As Well

The use of water on the *outside* of the body is a lot better and more widely understood, so probably needs little attention here. Yet a thorough daily bath, cleansing the body pores for both breathing and excretion, is helpful for those who want to live the full life.

Some alert parents point out that bathing can be expensive. That is true. It also can be inexpensive. In our home we take sailor showers—a technique I learned in the jungles of New Guinea where a shower, by necessity, consisted of a gallon can with holes in the bottom, hung just above my head from a tree: one gallon to get wet and suds up, and another gallon to get suds off. Sailors have to do it on ships where water is in scant supply. And we did it by necessity in New Guinea. If you apply the same principle in your bath or shower, you can cut your heat and water costs to far less than half, often saving several hundred dollars yearly for a normal family.

If you find that your children think they are deprived with such a procedure, take them down to some of the shacks across the tracks and let them see how some of their friends get along there. I remember well how as children we made out as best we could in the summer, much like we did in New Guinea. In the winter we all took our turns in the round galvanized tub near the wood stove. We had only so much money to buy coal or wood, and all the water had to be hauled in from the pump down the path by way of the back door. So mother and our little sister had their baths first; then we older boys followed in the same water, except for a little extra hot water from the tea kettle on the stove to warm our tub. We then stepped over into a barely lukewarm tub to rinse.

It is wise wherever possible to finish off with a quick cold shower or rub to close the pores and retain body warmth as well as to stir up circulation—one of our best of all preventive measures against disease. Whether inside or out, warm or cold, don't neglect the fullest use of water.

To everything there is a season, And
a time to every purpose under heaven.

Ecclesiastes 3:1

13

The Five R's—I: Rest, Recreation, Recuperation, Regularity, and Relaxation

During my tour with the U.S. Army in Milne Bay, New Guinea, during World War II, I was assigned for a period as commander of the Rotation Detachment and Casual Camp. Among the many who came through our command were men from the battlefront who were being sent to the rear, or sometimes home, for "R & R"—rest and recuperation. It was then that I discovered that *The Five R's* of this chapter were difficult to separate. If you discuss one, you in a sense are discussing all. We divide this topic into two chapters only for readability.

When one is recovering from any problem—whether it be overwork, stress, illness or surgery, traumatic experience, drug abuse or even boredom—we think of it as *Recuperation.* Yet each of us needs recuperation periodically, even daily, from the "cares of this life." Recuperation involves *rest, relaxation* and the kind of *recreation* that indeed re-creates. It also involves *regularity* because we often get ourselves into problems because we do not face the reality of natural biological rhythms which are an integral part of our life.

Since all of these are so intertwined and dependent on one another we decided to put them all together as a package, so to speak, because they all rebuild, rejuvenate and reorganize our lives. And in combination with the other health principles that God has given, these Five R's help to restore the image of God in us, which is His greatest desire.

Regularity

One day our secretary detected a special note of panic and female desperation on the other end of the line when she lifted the receiver. So instead of handling the call routinely, she called Dorothy to talk to the distressed lady. After asking a few questions, Dorothy had the message loud and clear. Here was a mother of five children, a dedicated Christian, who had just about decided that her family would be better off without her and she was ready to do away with herself. Utterly exhausted, she was frustrated with her efforts to do all the good things she thought she should but couldn't do. She obviously needed the Five R's, and quickly.

Dorothy made some emergency suggestions about eliminating certain things that were unnecessary and getting on a simple schedule. She extracted some commitments which involved the mother's first getting the cooperation of her husband and her children as helpers instead of hinderers. This included getting to bed early and having regular, consistent meals. Dorothy also requested that she have her husband call; she feared that he might not know the seriousness of the situation.

Her husband did not call back, but in about three days the mother *did*—jubilant over what a change had already taken place in her family. She realized that they had "a ways to go," but her husband had already adjusted his schedule. The family, including the children, had decided on 1) an early, light supper, 2) an early bedtime, 3) a substantial, early breakfast, and 4) a reasonable consistency. Despondency's dark clouds were already fading over the horizon.

One of the most common physical problems of women today is fatigue which can result in depression, irritability, impatience, and emotional outbursts. In general women who have families are self-sacrificing and in trying to handle all they think they should, they cut their sleep, nutritional needs, and anything to save time. Workaholic men do the same thing, but the reckoning eventually comes.

In counseling of all kinds, we have probably never found a simpler or more common single solution for marriage and family problems than to work to improve the regularity and basic lifestyle of the family. It is a part of God's ideal plan for us and it involves every part of our lives. The more nearly we cooperate with Him in His loving desires for us, the better "all things will work together for our good."

Unfortunately, few of us understand the need for regularity. We would rather do "what comes naturally"—often interpreted as "eat when you feel hungry," "sleep when you feel sleepy," and, in short, "do what feels good or convenient." Yet our God is the God of nature, and nature does not function in that way. Irregularity does not fit into His plan. Everything He created operates in perfect order.

Our Creator set in motion the solar rhythms of day and night, the lunar tidal rhythms, and the cycles of seasonal change which control our world. Astronomers can accurately predict the performance of these natural forces. They have not deviated in all of recorded history. Such widely varied creatures as fiddler crabs, salmon, and brown bears have distinct rhythms of activity. So do our bodies.

Yet, rather than being in tune with our natural environment, we have largely designed our activities on the basis of economic efficiency or convenience, at genuine risk to our health.[1]

One commonly recognized human rhythm is the monthly ovulation and menstruation cycle in women. In fact, each body system has a cycle and, though independent to some degree, is synchronized with the other systems. The relatively new phenomenon of jet lag has brought about more recognition and research on the effect of human lifestyle on these vital body cycles.

Circadian (Daily or Day-Night) Rhythms

Continued crossing of time zones in air flight in one instance landed an executive in the hospital with all the symptoms of a heart attack. Yet many travelers are not aware that such flights not only disrupt the internal clock but also impair mental alertness and physical energy. They even modify pulse, respiration, cell division, and brain waves; they interrupt monthly hormone levels and ovulation, and yearly cycles of cell replacement and reproduction.

But you say that this would not apply to you because you do not travel by jet airplane or perhaps any other way. Irregular hours *at home or on the job* and late night hours can do the same thing to your system. Research shows, for example, that rotating shift workers make more mistakes than workers on a regular daytime schedule. Doctors who are on duty between midnight and dawn make twice as many errors when reading such test results as electrocardiograms, nurses are more likely to dispense wrong medication, train engineers tend to miss more warning signals, and truck drivers have more vehicle accidents without any other vehicle involved at night. Because the crew involved in the 4:00 A.M. Three-mile Island nuclear accident in 1979 had been rotating weekly through night-evening-day shifts, a mistake precipitated by such disregard of body rhythms could easily have been a factor.[2]

One would naturally assume that even though the normal sleep-waking cycle is disturbed, body systems will all adjust simultaneously in a brief time—perhaps with a relaxed weekend. On the contrary, experimental studies indicate that even though body temperature adjusted almost immediately, excretion of some hormonal byproducts was not completely synchronized for five weeks and potassium excretion did not adjust appreciably for the entire experimental period.[3]

Sleep

I learned something about sleep and rest from a surgeon who was one of the most efficient and long-lived I have ever known. I learned to know Harry Willis Miller, M.D., by writing his biography for Harper & Row.[4] Giving up a substantial inheritance at the turn of the century to go to China as a medical missionary, Miller was once described by *Reader's Digest* Senior Editor Clarence Hall as possibly the greatest physician of modern times, "easily in a class with Albert Schweitzer."

One of the world's great diagnosticians, Dr. Miller was consulting or personal physician to such notables as William Jennings Bryan, Alexander Graham Bell, four U.S. presidents, and such rulers as Generalissimo and Madame Chiang Kai-shek, Madame Sun Yat-sen, Chou En-lai, and famed Manchurian Marshall Chang Hsueh-liang whom Harry Miller rescued from opium addiction. He was also the father of modern goiter surgery who reduced thyroid surgery fatalities from more than 50 percent to less than 1 percent.[5] And he personally established twenty-one hospitals around the world.

He was virtually the sole inventor of modern soybean milk which has saved the lives of millions of infants and others here and over-seas—originally in China where dairy cows were few.

He was already well into his eighties when we wrote *China Doctor,* and he walked with lighter step than many men half his age. One of the most important lessons he taught Dorothy and me con-cerned sleep and rest. Even in his eighties he normally slept no more than five or six hours until he died at age 97! We still need more sleep time than he did, but we asked him how he did it and still maintained his abundance of creative energy at his advanced age.

Here is his recipe: First, he lived an abstemious life, eating lightly and regularly of good food, and getting an abundance of exercise—which relieved the need for larger amounts of sleep. Second, he maintained that a short nap of fifteen to twenty minutes at midday was worth two or three hours at night, and third, he insisted that sleeping time before midnight was worth at least twice as much as the time in early morning.

I was reminded of this years later at an international medical meeting in West Germany where I was lecturing with Professor Gunther Hildebrandt, world authority on circadian (body) rhythms. He showed how a person can avoid stress, ill health, and earlier-than-normal death, by following the early-to-bed-early-to-rise wis-dom of the ages. He verified that sleep in the early hours of the night is worth at least two to three times such rest after midnight.

For Efficiency

This helped me to understand how old Dr. Miller could rise and go to work at three and four in the morning with little or no fatigue. It also tells how any normal person can almost double his daily efficiency, particularly students who are in high school or college. They can add three or four hours to their actual work or study time by going to bed early.

When I was vice president of a medical university, some of our faculty and medical students determined that the time before breakfast offers three to five times the efficiency of the hours after supper. Not only is the phone quiet, but the body battery has been recharged by a night of rest. It gives powerful support for the electrical currents required by the brain for ready learning. Since the stomach is empty, the body's supply of blood is available to the brain. Many a medical and law student has discovered this truth and has been able to carry on heavy studies while maintaining a job, or has lifted his grade-point average substantially.

This, of course, is not a new idea. There are many proverbs and bits of doggerel that testify to its age and wisdom. For example, "The early bird gets the worm," and "Early to bed and early to rise makes a man healthy, wealthy, and wise." This is true among nearly all the top executives we know. They are often at work at the home or office before most of their employees get out of bed.

For Control

Well-rested children and adults are more likely to be self-controlled, patient, cooperative, optimistic, and productive. Normally they are not so cranky, irritable, critical, willful, and lazy. On the average they will enjoy much better health and incur less medical expense. They will be better workers, and live longer with fewer headaches and less pain. At home, at school, and on the job, they will cause fewer discipline problems.

Ordinarily you will alternate between active or REM sleep, and quiet or NREM sleep. Sleep authorities have found that in the first phase there is rapid eye movement (REM) under your eyelids— the time when it is suspected that dreaming is more likely to occur. After an hour or two of REM, you are likely to slip into non-rapid-eye-movement (NREM) sleep which will move from near-wakefulness to a quiet sleep and then into a deep, slow-brain-wave sleep.

For Refreshment

As you grow older, you may tend to have sleep that is not so sound as when you were young. However, 1) a light fruit and grain supper (or no supper at all), 2) a brisk walk or other full-body exercise, and 3) a lukewarm shower followed by 4) a quiet time with your God (with cares of the day set aside), will set the stage for sound sleep for a normal, healthy person. A time to sing and read together is great for family togetherness, especially when it is followed by hugs and kisses, and for younger children, a tucking into bed. All this is conducive to sound, happy sleep.

And don't forget to encourage each of your family to make everything right before you go to sleep: *Don't harbor ill feelings toward anyone,* especially in your family.

Don't take hot or cold showers just before bed time, for they are stimulating at an hour when your body craves rest.

All of us have had sleepless nights, usually after times of stress or grief or unusual excitement. The solution should not generally be sleeping pills; they are only crutches. Rather, look at the causes— stress or grief or excitement—and deal with those problems yourself or with the help of others, and always with the sweet peace that God promises you if you stay your mind on Him.[6]

Some need more sleep, some less. If you get to bed early, you will certainly be among those who need less. If your children seem to need a great deal more than normal, have them checked by your pediatrician or family physician. It may be that you have lazy children. Don't let them lie in bed. Give them some responsibility, something to do, preferably with you. Don't permit indolence; it is not a good substitute for sleep, not if you are seeking to build sound character in your children.

Satisfying Sleep

Of course a number of factors enter into satisfactory sleep, in addition to time of day and length of rest. Again, *quality* of sleep will be influenced by the time, size, and quality of evening meals, kinds of activity and conversations just before bedtime, and the amount and quality of exercise during the day. Light evening meals, preferably consisting of rapidly digestible foods such as fresh fruit and grains, happy relationships at bed time, and adequate large muscle exercise during the day will have a lot to do with the soundness of yours and your children's sleep, and the quality of your life when you arise.

Sleep dominates the lives of infants during their first year and that is the time to establish good sleep habits. Although their sleep requirements diminish as they grow older, children usually do much better in developing self-control and happy dispositions if they have an hour or so of naps as late as six or eight years of age (as well as a regular, early, and consistent bedtime). As Dr. Miller pointed out, a midday nap, even if only for fifteen to twenty minutes, is a great pickup for tired and harassed mothers, particularly during their monthly time, during pregnancies, and at menopause. Fathers too!

One physician friend vowed that he was a "night person."

"Everyone, almost, thinks he is a night person," I joshed him. But he was adamant. He observed that if he moved his home from the eastern U.S. time zone across the country to the western time zone, he would quickly adapt to getting to bed three hours later, for 9 P.M. is three hours later in Portland, Oregon, than it is in Portland, Maine.

But the doctor—and he is a *very* good one—failed to realize that the body rhythms are like the rhythms of the tide or the moon. Your body rhythms relate to the time the sun goes down and the night sets in *wherever* you are. You can't beat them by simply moving two or three time zones away.

Most of the sleepless people with whom we have counseled have an identical excuse: "I am a night person." The phenomenon of "night persons" is largely a product of the electrical age. A century ago, and as recently as fifty years back when there was no electricity in many homes, the main night people—other than those who had to work at night—were prostitutes and their clients!

Some ministers insist that all human beings are night people, in the sense that by nature we are creatures of darkness until called into His marvelous light. Being late night persons is obviously not God's idea. His Son was an early morning person. Mark (1:35) describes the Savior's routine: "And in the morning, rising up a great while before day, he went out, and departed into a solitary place, and there prayed." Christ, who invented body rhythms, believed in getting a good start on the day when the body battery was recharged and His mind was most vigorous.

Dr. Hildebrandt verified in his lecture on body rhythms that anyone who violates the rhythms takes a risk. When asked about those who work late shifts or who change shifts which alter sleep schedules, he declared that such programs are contrary to body rhythms. Requiring regular or periodic late bedtime hours leads without doubt not only to irritation, impatience, and other personality problems, but also *on the average* to more frequent illness, more likely neurosis, and earlier death.

Anything that can improve yours and your children's disposition will give a substantial boost to family control, to the prevention of behavior problems. Sleep should not be overemphasized to develop lethargy and laziness. Managed with common sense, it is one of the most faithful servants at your command for personal success, family happiness, and control.

Rest That Recreates

A plan for rest was established at Creation when God finished His work in six days and rested on the seventh—not that He was tired as we are tired, but because He scheduled rest for our needs and as sort of a birthday celebration for His creation. The week is unrelated to any natural phenomenon in our universe, yet has survived intact to this day. It was arbitrarily chosen because, as sociologists have repeatedly observed, it fits our physical and mental needs—a safeguard against overwork, stress, and cares of this life— providing a change of pace, a rest from the routine of the six days of work, and a time for meeting in special dimension with our Maker.

Men have repeatedly tried to break this cycle by calendar changes or laws. During the French Revolution, I am told, the revolutionaries tried to stamp out everything connected with religion, so instituted a ten-day week with one day in ten for rest. It seems that the plan was dropped because of confusion and its disastrous effects.

Something similar happened in Great Britain during World War II when, to increase war materials production, the work schedule was set at seventy-four hours a week. Soon there were more accidents and spoiled work, loss of morale, absenteeism, irritability, and restlessness. When management reduced the week ten hours, much of the problem was decreased and production was equal. But when they cut back to 48 hours, production went up 15 percent. Subsequently, Great Britain instituted a law requiring one day of rest each week and two weeks of vacation each year. They rediscovered that God's principle, "Six days shalt thou labor," was best.

Vacations

For some reason there are people who seem proud "never to take a vacation." Perhaps they feel guilty for relaxing, but obviously they are not reasoning correctly. When Christ and His disciples were so busy they scarcely had time to eat, He said to them, "Let's get away from the crowds for a while and rest."[7] Of course, any change of activity may be restorative as long as it is pleasant and not overdone.

Dorothy often quotes a saying she learned as a child but never knew its source. It had more meaning when she learned to knit, for it went, "Sleep knits up the raveled sleeve of care." The same is true of any legitimate time for earned rest. Obviously, there is no excuse for laziness. The Bible also has counsel for that. In any case, all forms of rest, whether a weekend or extended vacation, should revive one physically, mentally, and spiritually. A long drive across the country in a short time, for example, is not what we are talking about. Such a trip would probably leave one more tired than when he started.

Solomon summed it up neatly when he wrote, "To every thing there is a season and a time to every purpose under heaven."[8] If we can learn this lesson of temperance and trust in God, the Five R's will work out very well.

Blessed are you . . . whose princes eat
at a proper time—for strength and not
for drunkenness.

Ecclesiastes 10:17, NIV

14

The Five R's: Part II

Ralph Waldo Emerson, the American poet, was offered a beautiful, fresh, red cherry between meals. Pointing to his stomach, he
answered, "Why should I start all this delicate machinery over
again for that little cherry?" He wrote (along the lines of Ern
Baxter) that "The years teach much which the days never know."
Both research and common sense suggests that he was precisely
on target with the cherry and with the years.

God has promised a blessing for balance and regularity in our
eating habits when He says, "Blessed are you . . . whose princes
eat at a proper time—for strength, and not for drunkenness." Eating
as sensual indulgence is a habit that is often established practically
at birth when little ones are fed for indulgence rather than need:
Parents fail to provide the example and control which infants have
not yet developed and then wonder why their children grow without
learning *self*-control.

Regular Meals

First, *appetite* is far different from *hunger*—which has a physical
basis but is often imagined. Appetite is a desire of your mind, a
learned response, which you must keep under control lest it control

you. In 1 Corinthians 9:27 the apostle Paul said, "I keep under my body and bring it into subjection." Evidently appetite is important to God or He would not have made it the first test of Adam and Eve in the garden. Satan devilishly tried to prove it a stumbling block to Jesus in the wilderness. And you can see its depredations all around you these days.

Just as your body has other natural rhythms already described, so it has an orderly system of digestion. The glands in your mouth, stomach and intestines, your pancreas, liver and gall bladder all go to work systematically—each depending on the other in a cycle of exercise and rest like all organs of your body.

If, at the beginning of a meal, the cells of your salivary glands were appropriately stained and examined under a microscope, you would see them filled with enzyme granules. During the meal the process of chewing depletes the enzyme supply. Three or four hours later, the cells again would show that they have been refilled. Then, if you want the best of digestion, they need rest before your system goes to work again.

In the same manner the gall bladder serves as a holding pocket for bile, concentrated three to tenfold, that is made by the liver between meals to emulsify the fat in our food.[1] This is done so that the enzymes can work on it and also digest the protein and starch.

One of the reasons between-meal snacking causes problems is that it depletes the body's digestive juices and makes them scarce at mealtime. Your digestion then is incomplete or delayed until the organs recover their supply, and fermentation and a fatigued digestion system are your reward. Though much more complicated, snacking is like adding uncooked food periodically to a pot of food after it has been cooking for a while.[2]

A method which has been used repeatedly to study the functions of the digestive system is a series of X-ray photographs. If you are given barium-sulphate suspension along with your meal, the shape and contents of your stomach and colon can be shown. X-ray specialists have seen pictures of thousands of stomachs and report that after a normal meal the stomach should empty in about three to five hours, depending on the type of food eaten. Then your stomach should be allowed to rest before starting the process again, making the interval between meals at least five or six hours.

Between-Meal Eating

Interruption of your digestive cycle has been shown to increase your stomach-emptying time significantly. For example, in one experiment which has been replicated several times, five subjects were given a normal breakfast and it was established that the stomach would be emptied of that meal in four and one-half hours.

A few days later the same meal was given, but one individual had an ice-cream cone two hours later. This increased the emptying time to six hours. When a peanut butter sandwich, a piece of pumpkin pie with a glass of milk or a half slice of buttered bread every half hour—without any lunch—was given to three of the subjects, they all had undigested breakfast in the stomach after nine hours. The last person had two chocolate candy bars between breakfast and lunch and two more between lunch and dinner. In this case more than half the breakfast remained in the stomach *after thirteen and one-half hours!*[3]

Snacking at any time of the day or night is a great American custom. Some have even thought it *necessary* for young children, pregnant women, and hypoglycemics. But there is a significant difference in this "supposed" need and what is really good for you! If you reasonably follow the principles of regularity throughout this chapter, yours will be a health reformation.

Snacking between meals causes no end of distresses. It brings on overweight because of excess calories including sugar and fat; it impairs digestion; it may deplete the stomach's hydrochloric acid—which is one of your two major protein digesting enzymes; it disturbs sleep; digs tooth cavities; induces hypoglycemia; it produces possible malnutrition from empty calories; and it promotes abnormal behavior and decreased mental and physical efficiency.

We particularly mention the problem of clearer thinking and greater muscular strength here, because blood is always channeled from the muscles and brain to the digestive organs when food is eaten. Your disposition is influenced because the regular rhythm of your digestion is disrupted. The net result is food spoilage, gas, heartburn, and a heavy, distressed feeling, sometimes wrongly interpreted as hunger. Then you solve it by spending your good money on antacid "friends."

Breakfast Time

Start with a Good Breakfast. You've heard this admonition many times. There are good reasons. For example, after identifying the cause of irritability and inattentiveness in unfed youngsters even the first thing in the morning, some schools have instituted breakfast programs at school. Negative effects of poor breakfasts are noticeable also in the work place where they are seen in reduced work output and efficiency, fatigue, and proneness to accidents.

Some well-publicized research was done at the State University of Iowa called the "Iowa Breakfast Study," which concluded that an adequate breakfast makes you more productive during the late morning hours, less subject to fatigue, and quicker in reaction time. Students also showed better attitudes and higher academic attainment.[4]

But you say you are just not a breakfast person! Or you simply can't eat so early in the morning! Why? It's probably because you did something wrong last night. You may have either had a late snack after having eaten plenty at supper-time or eaten too much too late, or both. You likely followed this by reading or watching TV—requiring the use of little or no energy.

Your digestive process was not complete before bedtime, so your stomach, small intestine, large intestine, liver, and gall bladder had to keep on working, only not as efficiently as before. All of your systems have been slowed down during your sleep, but they could not rest until their job was done. They need rest just as much as your muscles, eyes, and brain. So in the morning you pay the price: Your digestive system is exhausted and bleary-eyed. It can't, without protest, face another task so soon.

Your body organs need about nine to twelve hours at night without any work at all—a fast, if you please. And the morning meal is the time to *break* that fast. If you have eaten a light supper— preferably of grains and fresh fruit—or even better, no supper at all, you will be hungry for breakfast, which should be your largest meal. When the interval is not long enough between the completion of one digestive process and breakfast, the stomach simply rebels.

If you consistently do the right thing at night, your stomach and you will be ready to eat like the proverbial king. One-third to one-half of the calories for the day should be eaten then, putting the fuel in *before* the day's journey, not *after*. And what a precious time to have the family together at the dawn of your day. It is a golden opportunity for worship and prayer that God may set a hedge about them all before everyone goes his way. A good breakfast also gives everyone a sense of well-being, a better disposition, enough energy to work accurately and efficiently, and decreases the desire to eat between meals or to overeat later in the day.

Then what should you have for a hearty breakfast? Start with two or more fruits, at least one of which is raw, probably citrus for Vitamin C, if possible, but preferably not juice. Whole fruit is worth twice the money. And apples are probably the best all-round fruit. Then plan a main dish along with whole-grain bread or toast and a spread such as avocado, olive or nut. For a main dish we like cooked cereal best—steamed brown rice, oatmeal, millet, mixed grain cereal in different combinations, such as triticale, barley or rye flakes. We add chopped dates, raisins, and sunflower seeds or nuts before or after serving and use soy or nut milk or skim milk which preferably has been boiled.

Sometimes we make a big batch of whole grain waffles and freeze some for later use. We top these with different kinds of unsweetened fruit rather than syrup or jam. Dorothy also makes her own granola with a variety of grains, nuts, seeds, and dried fruit. Sometimes we add sliced bananas or other fresh or home-canned sugar-free fruit. What a feast! Sometimes we say it's like eating all dessert!

One year when Dorothy taught part time in the same school our children attended, and we all left home together in the morning, we had our main vegetable meal for breakfast—baked potatoes, beans, vegetables, salads or whatever. We took sandwiches and fruit for lunch and just had fruit for supper. With the right planning and an automatic oven or microwave, it is quite practical, especially if one or more of the family is on a typical day-time work or school schedule and you really want to get on the best possible program.

You will notice that we indeed had lunch like a prince and supper like a pauper. The ideal for supper is just fruit or nothing at all, but if needed, add only something like whole grain crackers, crisp sticks or zwieback (twice-baked bread) with no butter or margarine. This digests in a couple of hours and early enough to complete the digestive process before bedtime.

Dorothy began her own two-meal-a-day program along with no between-meal snacking while she was in college to avoid the weight problems which some of the other girls suffered. When food is of the right quality, it is almost impossible to gain too much weight on the two-meal-a-day routine. Though we always had light suppers, the children and I joined her in making them still lighter or nothing at all when I approached age forty and noted a few extra pounds. Besides, by then I had also recognized some very great advantages of the idea—no dinner for Dorothy to prepare, no dishes to wash, and a dream-free, tranquil night's sleep.

We try not to make too many exceptions, yet neither do we want to impose our lifestyle on others. When we need to adjust for evening social occasions or for other reasons, we plan ahead by omitting or cutting down on our lunch and eating lightly of what is served. Even at occasional conventions where hotel group-dinners are involved, I ask the maitr d' for fresh fruit plates instead of the usual vegetables and meat. We found that most hotels are very gracious about substituting.

We started this plan in Chicago when my board chairman, W. Clement Stone, hosted us at a series of $1000-a-plate fund raisers. A waiter at the Conrad Hilton was disturbed because we left our beautiful steaks untouched. When we told him we were vegetarians, he scolded, "Why didn't you tell me?" Since then, many of our table companions have also chosen the delicious fruit salads which they once envied. One even sent his steak back and asked for a salad like ours, remarking that he "never did like these heavy night meals, but didn't know there was any recourse."

Recreation That Re-Creates

Gardening is for fun, food, family activity, savings, exercise, and pride. What seemed a lost art for the average family a generation ago, has come back into style. A 1982 Gallup poll states that more than forty-two million homes have vegetable gardens and produce $18 billion worth of food—with a return of about ten to one on an average investment of seed, fertilizer, water, and pesticide.

So perhaps the greatest, most constructive exercise of all is gardening. It is strange how we will hire someone to mow our lawns, or buy a tractor that we can sit on, and then go out running on the road for exercise. Gardening offers an extra dimension of inspiration as we put the seed into the ground to give its life that others might have theirs. The spiritual context of gardening is unmistakable as we cultivate, weed, fertilize, prune and, finally, harvest. Children love these lessons if learned *at your side* in the garden.

If you do mow your own large lawn as we do ours, try *pulling* your mower instead of pushing it. Pulling is much easier for the large areas, and is said to place less strain on your heart.

Of course, if one counted time at the earning potential of the gardeners and the market value of the land, the economic benefit would not be so great, but from a practical viewpoint, the advantages are unsurpassed. Also many modern gardeners are using compost for soil enrichment which also practically eliminates a need for fertilizer. At least this is our experience with a three-year-old virgin-soil garden plot. Somehow there seems no comparison with the flavor and quality of fresh-picked corn, squash, green beans or tomatoes—with store-bought items.

Exercise

Dr. Paul Dudley White was once helping some of us set up a pilot program in Stoneham, Massachusetts, near Boston, to help smokers kick the habit. As President Eisenhower's physician, he regarded sound exercise as the best of recreation. On the agenda developed by Dr. Wayne McFarland and his colleague Elman Folkenberg was a combination of diet, liquids, warm and cold showers and . . . walking. Running, swimming, cycling, and other exercises were not discouraged as long as they did not interfere with the patient's health and comfort. But walking was available to all—to all who *could* walk, that is. And, although Dr. White was a great cyclist, he told us that walking "is as natural as breathing."

"But my doctor says I must have aerobics," protested one Stoneham smoker, in the 5-Day Plan to stop smoking.

"Aerobic exercise," answered the great heart specialist, "is any exercise that stimulates you to greater capacity and use of oxygen. And a good *brisk* walk does just that."

The American Physical Education Association has repeatedly touted walking as a sane exercise for all people. It is a safe, total-muscle-building, heart-supporting, organ-toning, lung-expanding, joint-lubricating, blood-circulating-and-vitalizing, bone-strengthening, weight-controlling, disease-preventing, nerve-quieting exercise, perhaps unmatched by any other of the aerobics. Dr. Bud Getchell insists that most people should walk, not run, if you want to stick with a fitness program. He notes that the dropout rate for high-intensity exercise like running is more than 75 percent after six months, while *more than* 75 percent of walkers keep on walking.[5]

In any event, the use of your legs in running, bicycling, and to some extent in swimming, acts as a second heart, as it pumps blood through your system. It "tones your innards," as one physician put it. It helps with elimination. It reduces pain for many who have arthritis. It certainly helps if you have hypertension or are in danger of a heart attack.

Dr. Kenneth Cooper of aerobics fame suggests seven things that exercise can do for you: 1) increase lung efficiency, 2) increase heart efficiency, 3) increase number and size of your blood vessels, 4) maximize your oxygen consumption, 5) improve muscle and blood vessel tone, 6) slow aging and physical deterioration and increase zest for life, and 7) help you to relax, reduce stress, sleep better, and have a happier outlook on life.[6]

With all the information available today on exercise, we don't propose to provide extensive counsel in this book. One of the simplest and best resources we know is *The Reader's Digest Guide to Family Fitness,* available as a reprint from Reader's Digest, Box 25, Pleasantville, N.Y. 10570. Yet we do suggest that you practice several activities and make them into habits: 1) Exercise enough daily to make you perspire and to breath deeply (See Chapter 17, *The Breath of Life*). 2) Walk as tall as possible wherever you walk—as if you had the top of your head tied to a sky hook. 3) Walk briskly and take reasonably long, relaxed strides as if you had some place important to go and intended to keep your appointment on time without strain. 4) Practice safety whether you are walking, running, cycling or swimming. 5) Exercise daily in the open air. 6) Keep your physical exercise and mental work in balance.

And there are several cautions which the wise remember: 1) Run only with experienced counsel, preferably from a physician who has experience in internal medicine (particularly for women). 2) Cycle only with good equipment, including sound brakes and a good quality helmet, and follow *all* traffic rules—even more carefully than when driving a car, for you are usually in greater danger. 3) Swim only when another experienced swimmer is near, and never, never attempt to hold your breath for long periods under water, lest you black out and drown. 4) Read carefully the American Red Cross manuals, usually available at your local library. 5) After strenuous exercise take time to cool down gradually; failure to do this releases a flood of hormones which have maintained your blood pressure to the peak required, and may cause fatal irregularities in your pulse. But exercise! Be regular! And you will rest, relax, and recuperate!

> . . . put a knife to thy throat, if thou
> be . . . given to appetite.
>
> *Proverbs 23:2*

15

The Battle of the Bulge

The famed battle on the French front during World War II probably required no greater insight and bravery than men and women face on their own fronts every day, and often through no fault of their own. I have been to war and know that in most cases the motivation to be heroes didn't take soldiers there. Most were in that war because they *had* to go, not because they *wanted* to go.

There are times when it takes far greater heroism to initiate a battle than to get caught in it. And how you react, once the battle is set, will tell how much of a hero or heroine you really are. Perhaps the most heroic of all are those who go all the way and "over the top" in the very personal battle for victory in appetite. We should encourage, not criticize them. Dr. James Dobson suggests that the problem of obesity, especially for women, "ranks near the top in the index of human misery."[1]

Some Like Them Fat

At the outset, we should also be careful about our assumptions on obesity. A few years ago when we lived in Michigan, a young couple asked if they could be married at our home which was on beautiful Lake Chapin. The nearly six-foot groom weighed in at an estimated 140 pounds. The bride, a registered nurse and a very bright young lady, weighed a declared 350 at about five feet, four inches. This made it very clear to me that 1) some people prefer fat people and 2) some fat people are self-possessed enough to be candid about their weight.

Most Like Them Trim

This, however, is not generally true, and therein lies one of the most common social and psychological problems of our times— an era of the skinny-bunny or of Miss Slim Trim. Yet we must practice the Golden Rule in trying to help others work out this problem, if and when they want help.

Overweight Whys

Many who are overweight or obese came by it because of parental ignorance or neglect, or failure in their environments. They find themselves in a battle because they were indulged into heavy eating while still small children, creating a handicap that lingers with them for life. They were taught to eat for pleasure more than from need. And still others were provided an inferior quality of nutrition at school. More on the sources of fat in Chapter 5, "Fat." But the problem is usually food-related, and we will treat that here.

Diet Cautions

In the first place, if you have a weight problem, you are faced with a smorgasbord—a smorgasbord of sure-fire ideas, as the Yellow Pages will readily testify. They all end in one of three ways: 1) disappointment, 2) illness or 3) success which comes from a change of lifestyle. Here the last is not the least; it is the *only* way to go if you are determined to go the way of truth.

To tack on Mrs. Skinny Bunny's Fast Diet Slow-down, or to pay out good cash for Miss Slim Trim's Tasty Candy Miracle Losses or yet Mr. Giant's Weight Lifter's Paradise, will almost inevitably be a mockery. It will be a miracle if you get any permanent satisfaction, and it is usually a total loss in the end. It will be total because you usually end up fatter and more frustrated—with paradise lost, more than your weight. Here is why:

Any dieting plan that does not address the way you eat and

sleep and exercise—and all the other factors laid down in this book—is at best only a partial solution and at worst an evil trick on you. Often you will need a physician's guidance, a professional who understands and upholds the principles of science as they mesh with Scripture. In all cases you will need a long-term maintenance program that not only guides you in what, when, how, and why you shall eat, but also in every constructive use of your body and mind.

The Key: Self-Control

You will anticipate the time when the novelty of your diet wears off. You will combine the voices of science and clinical experience, as we are trying to do here, with a genuinely happy spirit which finds you more concerned with others than yourself. Thus, whether you eat or drink or whatever you do, you will glorify God. And that which glorifies Him will bless you. Some may call it "behavior modification" or "assertiveness training" or "stress reduction" or "cognitive adjustment." But whether you are changing your behavior, asserting yourself appropriately, reducing your stress or learning how to reason well, the best goal is *self-control in the Lord.* He will be your help.

"But," you say, "if I even let down for a moment, my weight seems to go up twice as fast." Remember that your body adjusts as it takes in less food. Your metabolism—the rate at which you burn up calories—slows down. Your body actually gets along on less food. Thus, if you increase even to a diet that is normal for most people, it may be too much for you. Your now slow-burning fireplace can't handle all the fuel, and a lot of it just piles up. If you continue even a normal diet, be sure to increase the level of your physical activity.

Simple Hints

Also try chewing your food much longer, two or three times as long as before. The time in your mouth will be noted by the satiety center in your brain, and your mind and body will become satisfied with less food. Also, the food you do eat will taste much sweeter as you mix your saliva and its many enzymes thoroughly with your food. This in turn helps your food digest better: You will receive more energy while avoiding illness or distress.

When you go to market, stay away from the food sections which have tempted you to fatness. Don't buy when you are hungry. Don't fast to a degree that tempts you to override your good judgment and start eating "no-no's" just this once. Study the calorie charts and select foods which cooperate with your goals. Call them your friends. Put black *X's* over the others as your enemies. Psychology? Yes, the psychology of self-control.

When you sit down at the table, remember to 1) cut out free fats—butter, margarine, mayonnaise, fried foods, 2) limit your food to two or three varieties at a meal, and 3) try eating more food raw. And then get up after mealtime and take a half hour or so of moderate exercise. When such foods (as described in Chapter 11, "What Goes In Must Come Out . . . Healthfully") reach your digestive tract, fiber swells with water and traps sugar, slowing your body's absorption of carbohydrates.

Strong Motivation

"But," many have reminded Dorothy and me, "you obviously have little idea of the battle I have to fight." Maybe. Yet every day was a battle for Dorothy and me, even though we went on two meals a day thirty-five years ago, with no snacking allowed at any time. We vowed anew that we would keep ourselves neat and trim for each other. Each day's victory made the next day easier, until, with the cooperation of our children, then ages five and nine, we changed our lifestyle. And we have not had a day's hospitalization for anything but pregnancies in forty-eight years of marriage until Dorothy went in for hypertension from overwork and pressures of leading a national movement in education.

For one thing, we valued our marriage, and we took a lesson from a number of our friends and marriage counselees whose records of unfaithfulness or divorce derived directly from the obesity of husband or wife. More often it was the man who was turned off from a wife who had become increasingly heavy or sloppy. He now was quite naturally tempted to compare her with the slim-trims around him at the office, at the store or even at church. They reminded him of what she used to be, and he concluded that she was either dumb or didn't care. In any event she no longer was making a fair effort to maintain that early beauty of body and spirit that so attracted him to her. A number of times, of course, it was the wife who was turned off by an obese or careless husband. Yet some spouses do prefer more flesh!

Dr. Dobson's Quartet

Because Dorothy and I are still vulnerable from our lack of experience in fighting the battles of the bulge, we are picking up a few strands of the best conversation we have ever overheard about meeting the needs of those who are overweight. It comes from a James Dobson "Focus on the Family" interview with four women whose weight losses ranged from about 50 to more than 150 pounds, and who had managed not to gain back their lost weight. In each case the woman changed her lifestyle; in each case she focused less on self and more on God—whom she made up her mind to glorify. And in each case she was now an attractive, well-figured woman (by Dr. Dobson's personal estimates).

Kathy

The first of the four, Kathy, was a fatty from childhood. Her parents had not taught her to discipline her appetite. The odds are especially heavy against such an adult. She tried "all the diets" from high school on, but none brought permanent results. She had dresses of all sizes in her closet for use at any given point in one of her failed programs. During a pregnancy she gained, grabbing for the rationale that nursing her child would take off her weight. But it didn't happen. Thirty to forty pounds overweight after fifteen or so post-pregnancy months, she was "frustrated, out of control." Then she decided to lay her burden upon the Lord, and began the plan of "Overeaters Victorious." She lost thirty pounds in four months.

Neva

Neva Coyle, the founder of the plan, was a fatty from age 5. When Neva was 11 her mother was buying dresses for her, sized "Junior Plenty." Later she "starved into my wedding dress," glad that she had to wear it only once. Then 165–175 pounds, by the time she was mother of three she weighed in at 250. She tried desperately everything under the sun—pills, programs, clubs, and exercise spas and finally even intestinal by-pass surgery. The result was all kinds of complications: "blood clots, kidney stones, you name it, it was all there." Her children got used to her being "hauled out" of the house in the middle of the night to the hospital.

Finally she realized that she was killing herself, and recognized that, although a Christian, her experience with Christ was explicitly related to the fluctuations in the weight of her body. Then she decided to be completely Christ's, giving Him her total burden in the conviction that He had been tempted in all points as she was. It was no longer a matter of toying with God, praying at Him, but of casting her total dependence upon Him and moving with Him. What had been a sort of Christian humanism now became an experience of staying her mind on Him.

Nancy

Nancy, another of the four, sensed disgust in the eyes of her husband. She went into the bathroom to undress by herself and even avoided intimate relationships to keep from reminding him of her rolls of fat. A trip to the beach with her children was out. She felt ugly, hated herself, lost self-worth. Fortunately her husband responded faithfully. And even more fortunately, she found Christ.

The women told how they felt like second-class citizens. They were unable to wear designer jeans. They would sometimes get stuck in the turnstiles at the market! In one instance an airline attendant offered a woman an extension for a seat strap on the plane. They laughed grimly at how as high school coeds they would be asked for dates at senior proms, only to have their places taken by trimmer females. Referring both to precept and example, they agreed that the responsibility for poor eating habits ultimately rests upon parents from the date of each youngster's birth.

Lynn

Lynn, a pastor's wife, was 100 pounds overweight, yet was encouraged by her husband and children and even members of her church. But she knew that she had to establish some priorities. She was shocked finally at the idea that she was not looking fat simply because of a poor camera angle. And it was dishonest of her to try on size 18 dresses when she had to have 22's. One day when she was counseling courage and determination to other women of the church, she sensed that she was being a hypocrite. Then the big blow came the day she was faced by her son with a word of encouragement followed by the remark, "But, Mom, you're still a mighty big woman." In desperation she turned completely to Christ.

Giving Their Yoke to God

The women were often caught in cycles they could not handle. Many men have the same problem. When these women would argue with their spouses, they ate in frustration and anger. Then they got fatter and more guilty. In a tragic cycle, this drew ever more remarks from their husbands—their desperate husbands. Eventually, said one, she had to "pray every bite [of food] out of my mouth."

The four women realized that they were killing their marriages, their families, and themselves. Their death styles had to become lifestyles that were mastered by Christ. When they surrendered fully to Him and let their yokes become His burdens, they had great victories. This mastery will keep *you* trim as it did them, whether you have known obesity or not. We all want to be mentally, emotionally, physically, and spiritually attractive to our friends, our children, and our spouse. The best news of all is that the ideal diet suggested in this book will not leave you hungry! You can live on it forever!

Truly the light is sweet, and a pleasant
thing it is for the eyes to behold the
sun.

Ecclesiastes 11:7

16

Sunlight in the Temple*

One day a Jesuit priest-in-training was escorting us around Rome.
Not far from the Minerva Hotel where we were staying was the
Pantheon. Built in a large circle with bricks, mortar, and stone,
its great dome has no inside support whatsoever. But even more
remarkable in engineering, it has a great round opening in its center—
making it one of the architectural marvels of the world. This, he
told us, was significant to his Church, "with its meaning for the
holiness of Sunday—the day of the Sun."

Pantheon is from *pan* (all) and *theos* (god or gods)—the temple
of all gods. It was so constructed that the great opening made
way for the rays of the sun god, regarded by many pagans as the
god of gods. The great black-and-gold, four-posted altar that once
occupied the center of the Pantheon—and whose replicae may be
found as far distant as Montreal—now is the center of worship in
St. Peter's of Rome.

Through the ages man has looked to the sun for healing—spiritual,
mental, and physical. Its use by pagans should not obscure the

---

*For much of the information in this chapter we are in debt to Zane Kime,
M.D., a University of California scholar who practices in Auburn, California.
All documentation for this chapter, unless noted otherwise, will be found in his
book, *Sunlight*.

remedies in its rays. We, too, have our body temples which should be opened not only to the Son of Righteousness, but also to the light of the great planet which He endowed for our cure. I regret that I didn't know more of its hygiene before—an ignorance which many Christians share and which may be attributed in part to Christianity's aversion to sun worship.

Ancient Sun Worshippers

Nudity was of course widely practiced among the Greeks, who heralded *heliosis* or *arenation*—exposure of the body to the sun on the sand. Antyllus and Herodotus were among the Greek physicians who prescribed sunlight for everything from asthma and epilepsy to jaundice, bladder or colon problems and obesity. The Grecian beaches and Roman solaria were widely used for this different kind of "sun worship." Even today scientists find that pregnant women who sunbathe are likely to have an easier time in childbirth.

The sun is worth a great deal more respect than we give it, and gives us powerful reason to revere the God who made it. Dr. Richard Hansen lists a few interesting facts:

1. Only eight minutes is required for light to travel the 93 million miles to earth.
2. The temperature in the sun's center is estimated to be about 15–20 million degrees.
3. The sun is 1.3 million times bigger than the earth.
4. The sun is approximately 150 times as dense as water at its core.
5. Our earth intercepts only about one part in 2 billion of the energy radiating from the sun. This is just the right amount to keep us warm and give us the light we need.
6. The sun loses about 4,700,000 tons of its mass *each second* (as estimated from Einstein's formula). The earth receives 4.69 million horsepower per square mile.[1]

The Creator of our sun apparently attached enough importance to this bright orb that He had His prophets refer to it from Genesis to Revelation.

Modern "Sun Worshippers"

During the last century or two the sun has returned to popularity as a healer. At the turn of this century, in one of the most remarkable turn-arounds of modern medicine, physicians began taking tuberculosis patients out of dark recesses once thought to be necessary for remedy, and began exposing them to the sun's "miraculous" rays. We all know the happy result—the sharp decline which the sun and sound nutrition brought to "TB" infection. But unfortunately, with the advent of antibiotics, solar therapy has in the last 40–50 years been all but forgotten. We are too much in a hurry for the sun's more leisurely therapy.

As we have moved from the country to the city, we have also moved inside and away from the sun. Even our transportation plops us behind glass that largely cuts off the ultraviolet rays which the sun so generously offers. This almost certainly has a negative effect on both our mental and physical health.

Ultraviolet Light

Yet, says Dr. Zane Kime, now we know that even "single exposures of a large area of the body to ultraviolet light were found to dramatically lower elevated blood pressure. . . . to lower abnormally high blood sugars as found in diabetics, to decrease cholesterol in the blood stream, and to increase the white blood cells, particularly the lymphocytes which are largely responsible for the body's ability to resist disease."[2]

Ultraviolet light is a miracle worker. It increases the heart's efficiency, the glycogen stores in the liver, our resistance to infection, the oxygen-carrying capacity of our blood, adrenalin in our tissues, our tolerance to stress, our sex hormones, resistance of our skin to infections, our energy, endurance, and muscular strength. Finally, it improves our electrocardiogram!

Those who sunbathe or otherwise get out in the sun systematically will realize the above benefits and many more. They will find their heart rates decreasing and returning to normal more quickly after exercise. Their lungs will *absorb* more of the oxygen they breathe. Their breathing will become slower, deeper, easier. More on the desirability of this in Chapter 17, "The Breath of Life."

In a ten-week experiment at the University of Illinois, half of the men in a physical education class were given ultraviolet treatments. At the end of the period this group had increased their physical fitness by nearly 20 percent, while the other half scored only 1 percent improvement. The first group showed distinctly lower blood pressures, had only half as many colds, showed a greater interest in classwork, and had a better attendance record.

Sunlight and Heart Disease

With half of all Americans dying from heart attacks, stroke, and allied problems, we should be on the lookout for anything that will help. And there is much written in this book on ways of dealing with these problems. But sunshine complements all other suggestions. It even helps to reduce excess cholesterol.

In one study of thirty patients, a reduction of blood cholesterol was noted two hours after a *single* sunlight treatment. Other studies have replicated this research, some with much larger numbers of patients. Patients are often astonished. One lady, age 65, dropped her cholesterol count from 333mg/dl to 221 in four days, primarily with sun treatment. Her triglyceride count was reduced from 299 to 197.

In a sense sunlight becomes a natural insulin. It reduces blood sugar levels—which contribute to heart attacks, artery diseases, gangrene of the extremities, and many other problems. The light of the sun apparently helps the absorption of glucose (blood sugar) into the body cells for the storing of energy in the liver and muscles. For many diabetic patients exposed gradually and progressively to the sun, it has been found that sunlight has caused the sugar in their urine to decrease or disappear, with less craving for sweets.

High Blood Pressure (Hypertension)

The pressure on the arteries while the heart is pumping is *systolic*. When the heart is at rest, the pressure is *diastolic*. When these pressures run above 140/90, you are an endangered species. You may be under stress or eating too much of the wrong things or lacking exercise, among other things discussed in this book. Depending on the person and the cause, the pressures may be reduced by medication or by natural means.

One of these natural means is sunlight—which can have a profound effect in reducing blood pressure. Some patients have reduced their blood pressure as much as 40/20 after only a day or so of treatments. The Russians are now getting excellent results from sunlight at their resorts.

If there is any question about the use of sunlight, consult a physician who is familiar with this research. For example, those with dark skin (which is more impervious to sunlight) will have different requirements—and potential results—from those who have lighter skin. And you will do well to read Dr. Kime's book thoroughly for yourself.

Sunlight and Aging

Sunlight, oxygen, and polyunsaturated fats all play a part in the aging process. But this does not mean that you should stop breathing or stay out of the sun. Advertisers plug their polyunsaturates on television, radio, and in print. You will be tempted to believe that you cannot survive without them—much as proteins were overdone a generation ago.

Sunlight and Vitamins

There are a number of helps in avoiding this aging process: *Vitamin C* from natural sources such as citrus, strawberries, tomatoes, and dark green leafy vegetables. *Vitamin E* from whole grains, fresh vegetables, whole nuts, and seeds. *Vitamin A* from yellow, carotene-producing fruits and vegetables such as carrots, sweet potatoes, melons, squash, pumpkin, apricots, peaches, corn, bananas, and from dark green leafy vegetables.

Vitamin D, on the other hand, is now considered to be more a hormone than a vitamin. While you may derive it from a variety of capsules and pills, studies in England and Massachusetts have demonstrated conclusively that there is no *D* source like the sun! One researcher concluded that exposing a baby's face to sunlight for even a few minutes during the middle of the day, even in winter, would provide enough D to protect him from Vitamin D deficiency. So our conclusion is simple: more sunshine wherever possible, and fewer pills.

Sunlight and Infectious Diseases

Over a hundred years ago A. Downes and T. P. Blunt found that light could kill bacteria. They placed clear glass tubes of brown sugar water on a window sill, some in the sunshine, some in the shade. They noticed that those in the shade became cloudy, indicating bacterial growth, while those in the sun were clear. They decided then that sunlight and bacterial growth don't go together. From their discovery in 1877 there has been a progression of findings which assure us that sunshine is one of the greatest enemies of infectious disease. In experiments involving tuberculosis alone, it was found that surgery was 22 percent effective, medical treatment was 30 percent successful, and ultraviolet an astonishing 75 percent!

When we get this vitamin act together, the sunshine can wrap up the package and give you younger-looking skin and longevity. With the combination of sunlight and vitamins from natural sources, Dr. Robert Bradley, of *Husband Coached Childbirth* fame, insists that the "skin is more flexible, less brittle." All authorities on sunlight ask you to remember not to overdo a good thing. If you have any questions, see your dermatologist, geriatric specialist or family practice physician.

Sunlight and Cancer

No one seems to know the precise relationship between sunlight and cancer, although like the aging, above, they caution not to expose yourself too much too soon. It is believed that the sun may have an effect on your body if you have abnormally high cholesterol levels. The more fat you eat, the more likely you will develop cancer of the skin as well as of the breast and colon.

The effect of a combination of polyunsaturates and excess sunshine may be cancer formation. Dr. Kime notes that one way sunlight helps bring on skin cancer is that, with a high polyunsaturated fat diet, your immune system becomes depressed. Your body is then unable to stop the growth of cancerous cells. Even polyunsaturates alone can inhibit your immune system, but the wrong use of the sun, in combination, can accelerate the process. The growing danger can be seen in the statistics: Salad and cooking oil consumption, with the urging of "health-minded" manufacturers, has increased from 1.5 pounds per person per year in 1909 to about 25 pounds today. You are what you eat!

That brings us to a series of "ifs": If you eat *as natural a diet as possible* of whole foods, if you avoid any substantial intake of polyunsaturates (and preferably none), if you take your sun gradually, and if you do not allow yourself to become overheated, the sunlight will inhibit cancer rather than cause it.

Sunlight and Nutrition

The intimate relationship of sunlight and nutrition is well illustrated by the sun's producing of hormones and nutrients like Vitamin D. And you can conclude rightly from our previous discussion, that sunbathing is more likely to be hazardous for those who are on the Standard American Diet (SAD) with its surplus of fats, particularly when they do not have a balance of fresh fruits, vegetables, and whole grains in combination with a reasonable amount of appropriate exercise and rest.

Sunlight and Antibiotics

Strangely, antibiotics, so widely received and popularized during World War II, turned our society away from the sun. They were fast acting—just like many drugs today—and in the day of speed, why be bothered with anything so slow as sunshine? But now we are paying the price in new, more dangerous and resistant bacterial strains which future antibiotics may not be able to handle. Meanwhile the sun waits patiently in the wings to come on with its act when we have enough sense to signal its curtain call.

Whether the diseases are colds or flu, meningitis, tuberculosis or even cancer; whether they are airborne, waterborne or carried in other ways, we must open all avenues to the sunlight and welcome it as our most favored guest. Wherever possible, open your curtains, throw back your bed sheets daily, hang out your clothes periodically.

Keep your skin as clean as practicable, and let the sun get to it to divinely disinfect. Strengthen your immune system in any way you can; or should we say, don't do anything that will deter it! Build your blood with wholesome food and plenty of pure water appropriately ingested, and call, always call, sunlight to the rescue.

And finally, in this section, sunlight destroys CAMP. This substance, *cyclic adenosine monophosphate*, builds up in the lymphocytes in your blood so that they are unable to function properly and, for example, cannot destroy cancer cells or may otherwise depress your immune system. CAMP is increased by such stimulants as caffeine, theophylline, and theobromine—found commonly in coffee, tea, and chocolate. Their stimulating effect comes directly from their production of CAMP. Coffee and tea are said to be especially dangerous in this production, and they thus endanger your immune system. Fortunately CAMP is sensitive to light and sunlight destroys it.

Sunlight and Air

In Chapter 17 we show how sunlight electrifies the air, charging it with a high ratio of negative to positive ions. But air without sunshine is like beans without salt. They provide nutrition, but aren't nearly so much fun. And sunshine may be a principal reason why we are somehow surviving an air pollution dilemma which by all normal estimates should have had more of us dead 'ere this.

Sunlight and Psychology

Few rational people will deny the emotional lift that the sun brings. Solomon's words at the head of this chapter tell the story for nearly all of us. It is astonishing that modern medicine has ignored this great healer, and often keeps patients indoors when they should be outside.

It is such enlightened medicine that is being used at highly successful treatment centers like the institutes at Weimar, California; Hartland (Orange), Virginia; Hermosa, South Dakota; Uchee Pines (Seale), Alabama. This is highly professional and sterling-principled medicine that does not bow to expedient and limited drug therapy except where absolutely necessary. And it is endorsed and used by wise traditional doctors who have to stay by their more conventional practices.

Tinted eyeglasses often produce or abet abnormal behavior. Even the eating habits of fish are affected by unnatural lighting. And experiments have demonstrated that students treated with sunlight are more "wide awake" than those who are not. Sunlight helps keep in balance the stimulating and depressing nerve impulses.

Sunlight and Sexuality

We often hear conjecture these days about the early maturation of our youngsters. Some are certain that they are influenced by sexual talk, and that may be. Others suggest that their parents give them so little attention they have to grow up on their own.

And we know that excess protein is also blamed. But there is also another reason. Children who grow up inside their homes and schoolrooms tend to mature faster than those who can run freely out of doors. Children are naturally creatures of light and day.

Rats, on the other hand, are creatures of night. As long as they operate in the dark, they will mature normally. But when they are kept in perpetual day, their growth and maturity is accelerated, and they will not live as long.

The change in the age of maturity has been observed all over the world where we have kept our children more inside than out. Dr. Kime points out that J. S. Bach's choir boys of 1750 A.D. experienced voice change at age 18. Today the average age is 13.5!

There is clear reason for sunlight's influence: It stimulates glandular production when it passes through the eye into the brain, and when it produces hormones directly in the skin. The pineal "gland" in the middle of the brain is stimulated to produce hormones which directly affect the pituitary, adrenals, ovaries, and testes. The *melatonin* which the pineal secretes actually induces sleep and can change the brain wave pattern, stop the ovaries from ovulating, and even delay maturity.

The Unfortunate Nurse

By rare coincidence Dr. Kime reports on a young woman, then age 23, who, though not a blood relative, was family to us. From a distinguished, nationally known family, beautiful and normally energetic, she had studied hard to complete her nursing course in record time, and became so preoccupied with helping patients in a hospital that she had little time for herself. Some of us worried that she was overdoing. She was. But we did not know what to do about it. Nor did we know that she had not menstruated for over two years, and had been plagued with continuous diarrhea.

Yet Dr. Kime turned up this information in a routine physical examination, ascertained that she had been indoors most of the time, and prescribed daily sunbaths, beginning with short periods and extending to several hours. He also asked her to bare her neck of her long hair when she lay on her stomach, to permit the sun to reach her pineal gland at the base of her brain. Within two months she was menstruating again and her diarrhea was long gone.

Sunlight produces an estrogenlike substance in the skin which moves into the blood, elevating female hormones, and even more rapidly elevating hormones in the male.

When the pineal gland is destroyed, and with it its production of melatonin, animals have been found to be more susceptible to cancer. Most Americans by age 50 have calcified pineal glands, as compared with less than 10 percent in Japan and about 5 percent in Nigeria. These figures show a striking similarity to the incidence of breast cancer in these countries.

Sunlight and Obesity

Sunlight can even help obesity. The sun stimulates the thyroid gland. It in turn increases the body's basal metabolism rate, burning up calories faster. The sun also tones the muscles under the exposed skin. This burns more calories and encourages loss of weight.

Sunlight shares its blessings in other ways: It is a boon to arthritics, warming and loosening stiff, sore joints and bringing some relaxation. It is a healer of wounds (physical and mental), sores, ulcers, psoriasis, acne, certain skin cancers, and, according to some, it even stimulates hair growth.

Sunlight How's

But take care not to overdo it! Dr. Kime preaches what he practices. If you are light skinned, you usually must take greater care. The sun will work faster on you. In the summer it is better to sunbathe in the morning when the air is cooler. No overheating, please. At least move to the shade for a while or take a dip or a lukewarm shower. Feel free to sweat; it cools you and gets rid of body poisons, and even absorbs some of the sun's rays.

Sunbathe the year around by finding a corner out of the wind. And stay away from fats or oils under or on your skin, for they may stimulate the formation of cancer cells. If you decide to use a tanning lotion, be sure that it does not have fat as a base. And if you do not have sunshine available, do the next best thing: Purchase fluorescent tubes that produce ultraviolet rays with frequencies above 290nm. Mount them on the wall in a vertical position so that you can stand about two feet away, turning so as to expose all sides of your body.

And always wear protective glasses against these rays. Start with a minute or two, and gradually increase your exposure, so as not to burn. Dr. Kime warns not to install the light over your bed or table for horizontal treatments unless you have—and use—a timer, lest you doze off and become burned.

So much of our health depends upon our appreciation of sunlight and our determination to use it wisely. Although this is no theological coup, we can't resist quoting Proverbs 4:18 which combines with our early text to inspire us to accept the sun as a gift of God, appreciating the gift and worshiping only the Giver: "The path of the just is as the shining light, that shineth more and more unto the perfect day."

God breathed . . . and man became a
living soul.

Genesis 2:7

17

The Breath of Life

One day, during our tour of duty in Japan, I was called from
our college to visit a dying girl in the Kisarazu hospital. I was
not prepared for the scene. This lovely girl, a victim of advanced
tuberculosis, was literally gasping and choking to death. There
were only a few cubic inches of air space left in her lungs, and
without air she could not live. After a short talk with her and
prayer together, she began the sleep of those who await the resurrection. And I went home moved by two lessons: the beauty of
one who dies in her Savior, and the wonder of lungs filled with
fresh air.

Our need for air is more urgent than our need for water, just as
we need water more urgently than food. Deep breathing of good
air helps our blood to circulate freely, refreshes us and strengthens
every function of our bodies. There is nothing more relaxing than
a deep breath of fresh air, nothing that brings more immediate
serenity or induces sleep or excites the appetite and helps our food
more perfectly to digest.

Those Healthful Ions

Good, fresh air is made up of 78 percent nitrogen, 21 percent
oxygen and 1 percent argon, carbon dioxide, helium, and other

miscellaneous gases. We need not only fresh, clean air, but also negatively ionized air. The air, ideally, is charged with positive and negative ions, and the more negatively charged it is, the healthier it will be.[1]

This ionization occurs best in climates where sunshine and moving water are present. Waterfalls, the movements of the ocean and streams help the breakup of water droplets so good for fresh air.[2] And it is well known that smog—dirty air of any kind—decreases the concentration of these negative or "happy" ions in your oxygen.[3]

Animals reared in well-ionized air are found to learn twice as fast as those breathing ordinary air. The well-ionized atmosphere may provide a more relaxing environment.[4] The implications for astronauts cooped up in space and sailors in submarines are beyond the imaginations of some of us. But even more significant by their numbers are children in today's classrooms who have little sunshine and fresh air. Theirs is anything but the best of learning environments.

The more well-ionized oxygen you breathe, the less likely you are to have heart and artery problems, high blood pressure, diabetes, even glaucoma, cataracts, and cancer. By slightly increasing the oxygen concentration in your air intake—and therefore your blood—you decrease your cholesterol and tryglyceride levels and even hardening of the arteries may be reversed.[5] But if you increase the fat content in your blood, your oxygen intake will decrease, your red blood cells are more likely to be sticky and to "clump." Your blood will not flow freely through your fine veins.[6]

Air and Your Eyes

George Chen, ophthalmologist and preventive medicine specialist, tells of the slowing of the blood by this process even in the eye.[7] He notes that this can be clearly seen in microscopic studies. This explains at least partly how good breathing habits help prevent glaucoma and cataracts.

Breathing Cautions

Among the cautions in breathing are: 1) Avoid automobile and factory exhaust fumes, tobacco smoke, solvent fumes, and household cleaners which pollute the air; and 2) avoid hot desert storms such as you find in North Africa, the Middle East, and the western deserts of the United States. These tend to produce strong positive ions as in carbon dioxide, etc., which may last for a day or two. Third, try not to spend most of your time indoors.

Breathing Helps

Here are a few things to remember if you want the maximum breath of life:

1. Think lofty thoughts, as though every breath were in fact from heaven.

2. Breathe deeply. Practice taking extra draughts of air before you exhale—perhaps as many as ten quick breaths—then exhale promptly through your mouth. It will help if you think of breathing from your diaphragm—down at the bottom of your lungs—instead of shallow draughts from the top. Practice the idea of exercise such as walking up hill or running enough to bring you to your *second wind*—that point at which in heavy exercise you no longer feel out of breath.

3. Do not wear tight clothing which restricts this action. The tighter your dress or trousers around your waist, the less healthy you will be. Suspenders, now back in vogue, are best for support of trousers. We do not suggest that you should put on sackcloth, but simply to avoid restrictive, constrictive clothing if you want the freedom in breathing so crucial to good health.

4. Exercise regularly out of doors if possible.

5. Sleep with your windows open at night whenever possible, using more covers, if necessary. You can close your bedroom door to the warm rooms of your home to conserve fuel. Your breathing will be richer in negative ions.

6. Air out your bedding, and sun it also whenever possible, to avoid pollution from body odors and gases.

7. Eat a diet as low as practicable in fats, particularly animal fats, to facilitate the work of ions in smoothing the flow of your blood.

8. Spend as much time as you can out among trees. Pine trees are considered especially good medicine for your lungs.

9. You will be more comfortable if the air you breathe is neither too dry nor too moist. It may be necessary at times to use a humidifier in climates which are too dry or a dehumidifier in climates which are too moist.

Thou wilt keep him in perfect peace
whose mind is stayed on thee, because
he trusteth in thee.

Isaiah 26:3

18

Temperance, Stress, and Trust in God

In 1962 a lone Japanese man made a 94-day trip from Japan to San Francisco in a 19.1 foot sailboat. When he was asked how he was able to endure the isolation and loneliness, he made three significant explanations. First, he was determined to overcome all difficulties he might encounter; second, he used a compass faithfully to see that he was heading in the right direction; third, he had trust in his vessel because it had been designed by Japan's top boatbuilder, and he had watched to see that everything was carried out according to the designer's plan.

He had determination, direction, consistency, and trust. He had an orderly plan, avoiding detours, distractions, and discouragement. These set the stage for victory. His was a remarkable feat, but it doesn't compare with the ocean before you and me. Our navigation poses a much greater risk than his, and we need navigational help as well from the Master Designer.

Quieting Your Storms

All the sailor's trust was in his own strength and ingenuity—the sheer humanistic approach. But you can ask your Creator to quiet your storms as surely as He brought peace to the raging waters while resting in a fishing boat with His disciples that night

on Galilee—if you have the faith of a child in Him and His love
and guiding hand.[1] As long as the Bible is your compass, you
will not lose your way. Your trust will not be in a boat, but in
the Designer who knows all, sees all, is ever-present and all-powerful
and whose creations are perfect. To turn from His ways is, of
course, humanistic, too, especially for the Christian.

Stress is found in any experience which requires you to cope,
adapt or change in some degree. It can be either positive or negative,
and in this world there is no way totally to avoid it. Indeed, the
absence of stress physically and mentally, is death. You need it
for productivity and motivation. The amount of stress and your
response to it tells the tale of your life and how you live it.

Nutrition and Stress

Your diet has an explicit influence on your mind. It may encourage
a happy and peaceful life with a good attitude toward your friends
and family—or it may bring on impatience, stress, and even depression. And these negative feelings may range from mild to violent
or suicidal. Even so simple and common an experience as a heavy,
late supper will almost always bring regrets the next morning—
except that few seem to know the real reasons. "Mornings after,"
from food and drink, sometimes bring genuine depression.

On the other hand, *lack* of nutrition may be the cause of problems.
One woman was so panicky and depressed from her abnormally
low carbohydrate-reducing diet that she suddenly raced out her
front door to throw herself in the path of an oncoming car. She
was saved by an alert husband, who raced to overtake her and
abort her suicide attempt, and she recovered with some simple
changes in her diet. Another, thought by her psychiatrist to be a
hopeless schizophrenic, was brought around in a few months by a
nutritionally oriented family doctor who prescribed a conservative
diet.[2]

Intemperance and Stress

Intemperance often brings stress into your life. If you not only
overeat, especially at night, but also go to bed late, even normal
circumstances in the morning can be stressful for you. Though
much of the world's population is undernourished, some nutritionists

suggest that most of those who are adequately nourished are really *eating too much*. Our nutritional counselors have advised that in general, only hunger should be satisfied, not appetite, and maintaining the lowest weight at which your strength is still optimum is the ultimate goal.

Intemperance sometimes consists of very constructive activities—perhaps just too much of a good thing. For example, your work may be so fascinating and exhilarating that you have a hard time not allowing it to permeate every phase of your life—even your sleeping hours. Or there may be people, too many of them, all of whom are loved and lovely; or travel which is interesting and exciting keeps you on a perpetual high. Stress comes from too much of anything, good or bad, that keeps you from living a balanced life.

Though we have suggested moderation in a number of instances throughout this book and reminded you of your obligation to God with respect to your health, only you can do something about excesses in any line. To be temperate is to exercise self-control which is the quality needed if you are to successfully run the race and achieve mastery—for the incorruptible crown.

Personal Discipline

Carelessness, unnecessary dirt and clutter in the house, garage or yard do not promote peace; rather, they nearly always lead to strain, stress or ill health. Cleanliness, we were taught, is next to godliness. I recently had to warn a mother who was being taken to court for home schooling that she should clean up her act or I could not witness for her in good faith. Example is the best teacher always; such disarray was not teaching her children the right habits. They would be better off away from home, at school, unless she corrected her problems from basement to attic, inside and out.

Often you will hear people making fun of the Army. They laugh at its discipline, sneer at its sheer pickiness. But an army without this control would be no army at all. Of all the common denominators we have ever seen in the management of families and men, we know of none which works like order, service, and self-control, cradled in complete trust in the grace of Christ and the promises of God.

"Join the service" means giving of self. Such a gift means, first, self-control. When self is fully surrendered to the will of

God and the service of our neighbor—whoever he may be—stress no longer reigns. Our burden becomes our Savior's burden; our yoke is transferred to His neck. And this He is well able to bear.

Service and Stress

Service for others was central in the life of Christ. True love always brings compassion—the echo of heaven. If you are having trials, burdens you cannot bear, try visiting others who are aged or ill or who are having trials of their own. Have you ever visited a jail or prison or penitentiary? Try it sometime. Find from the counselor or your newspaper someone who is in trouble and work from there, usually with men helping men and women helping women.

If your children are becoming selfish and demanding, especially in their early years, take them out to a nursing home or pediatric ward or to families who are hungry. Watch their fussing and demands vanish and peace come to your home as they forget about their own needs, as they see the distress of others.

The Security of Regularity

In case tranquillity is not your habit, let us be very specific in regard to your own personal health: (1) How *regular* is your day? Regularity is such a firm law of nature that it won't be denied no matter how you try. You might reread Chapters 13 and 14, on the Five R's and reevaluate your biological rhythms, and especially read about pre- rather than post-midnight sleep. (2) Could your diet be out of control? Good quality fuel in the right amounts at the right time makes your machinery run better. (3) How about a hot and cold shower in the morning to give your day a good start with better circulation and fresh oxygen to your brain? (4) Are you getting daily exercise, preferably in the sunshine and fresh air? Recheck Chapter 13 and see what exercise does for stress. (5) Are you exposing yourself to stress which may be unnecessary yet at the same time becomes unavoidable as you watch TV violence and even stress-producing daily news which you could do without?

The Relief of Right Doing

Having done your part, you still have the best recourse of all. Along with the consciousness of right doing and the assurance of

God's approval, the knowledge that God is an operating partner in your activities not only promotes physical health but also provides great stability for the stresses of life. Such confidence is fortification against doubt, perplexity, and excessive grief which would otherwise sap the vitality and bring on nervous diseases. "Thou wilt keep him in perfect peace whose mind is stayed upon thee, because he trusteth in thee."[3]

The more you know about the sympathetic connection that exists between the mind and body, the more you will understand the significance of this promise of "perfect peace." When you learn to "trust," you unload on God. As you let Him carry your burdens, stress marvelously disappears.

Japan and God

In Japan, the post-World War II circumstances were sometimes so deplorable, even vicious, that one of our friends predicted we would last no more than six months. He predicted we would come home with a nervous breakdown. We stayed five years, and frankly never did think for a moment of the stress on a campus which, we were warned, at first was deep in debt, riven with disease, and with morale drained to its last dregs. But our dear friend, Wilton Baldwin, an educator without super-advanced degrees, who knew his God, taught us lessons of trust which became almost absolute. Once that surrender to God is made, stress is gone. It was one of the most precious periods of our lives.

I well remember reading Isaiah one day when our financial situation seemed hopeless. We had little or no subsidy as other colleges did, and yet had to pay off 17 million yen of debt. Then I found Isaiah 58. Read it! We were told not to mope or be discouraged, but to arise and shine, and follow as God led. Then all sorts of things would break loose. And they did. Sons of strangers did build our walls as Isaiah predicted: The brother of the Emperor came to our campus to give it credibility.

Donations flowed in. Our new campus industries flourished. As Isaiah promised, we sucked the milk of the Gentiles, and were ministered to by kings. We were out of debt and, though small, became an educational institution to be reckoned with in the Land of the Rising Sun. It was a miracle of God, and all without fearful stress.

Another way to look at temperance and stress is through eternal eyes. What are we doing here, anyway? Our citizenship is in heaven.[4] We are a royal priesthood.[5] We are joint-heirs with Christ, the King of kings and Lord of lords.[6] We are in fact kings (and of course queens) who are preparing to sit one day with Him on His throne.[7] It will ease a great deal of stress if we simply say, with our hands in Christ's, "I'm going to let You take care of this. It can't possibly last very long compared with eternity, and eternity with You is my goal."

God's Conditional Promises

This does not mean that we don't have anything to do. *All of His promises are conditional.* And that's the way it should be with an all-wise, all-powerful heavenly Parent. Look at Exodus 15:26. He will keep you well *if* you listen carefully to Him and do all He tells you to do. Look also at Deuteronomy 28:1–14: His blessings will come on you and overtake you, *if.* . . . And read 1 Samuel 2:30: He will honor you *if* you honor Him. And again, Proverbs 3:6: He will give you direction *when you acknowledge Him.* The fifth commandment[8] makes honor to our parents a condition of long life. In fact from Genesis 2 to Revelation 22, God's conditions are lovingly laid down like guard rails for our behavior.

Yet, *God does not hold us responsible for those things we do not know!* Your infants are not held eternally accountable for their actions. Until they learn to reason consistently, you, their parents, are responsible for them and in a sense are as God to them—in trust from their Maker.

Sane Psychology

I am a psychologist and could go on psychologizing for the rest of this book. And you would suffer. Man-made solutions are all around us. But God's solutions are simple, direct, and absolute. We have already told you about Psychiatrist J. T. Fisher and his evaluation of the Sermon on the Mount.[9] As he observed, it is one of the most remarkable treatises on mental health ever written or spoken. We have also reminded you of the Golden Rule—the essence of godliness.[10]

Dr. William Wilson, professor of psychiatry at Duke University in North Carolina, is a dear friend of ours and one of the sanest psychiatrists I know. I speak of sanity as something to be cherished among psychiatrists, because during World War II I found, as a medical personnel officer on General Douglas MacArthur's staff in Manila, that by far the largest number of specialists we sent home on medical discharge were psychiatrists who couldn't take the stress of the war zone.

Dr. Wilson himself was under considerable stress as a psychiatrist, trusting as he did in modern scientific theories of the mind. But he was not aware of his condition until one day a fellow physician-professor with a badly troubled mind mirrored Dr. Wilson's own fatigue and a life that seemed to alternate clutter with emptiness. With all his eminent skills Dr. Wilson could not find a solution for his sick client.[11]

Then one day he went on a week's wilderness canoe trip with his son's Boy Scout troop. He had not been a religious man, though as a boy he found peace in the forest and its streams. Now, from the ministry of the scoutmaster, the placid lake, and the trees, along with a rereading of Matthew 23, Dr. Wilson sensed that he needed a cleansing that only the God of the scoutmaster could offer. On that trip he found a new outlook on family and home—an altogether new experience for a man in a profession that had little use for religion. Even the hospital had a rule that no incoming patient could have a Bible. So Dr. Wilson kept his professional life separated from his spiritual experience.

Then one day a special case was brought to him—a drug-addicted physician. After two months of the usual treatment there seemed to be no progress. The desperate man pled with Bill Wilson. At that point, Dr. Wilson, who was also at his wits end to help his patient, finally related his own experience and said to him, "Pray. Just get down on your knees and pray. And don't get up until you've felt God in your life. . . ."

The next morning, vows Dr. Wilson, the addicted physician was well. And to this day prayer remains this Christian psychiatrist's most effective tool. "Now," he says, "I pray regularly for every person in my care" before, during, and after counseling sessions. "The power of prayer never ceases to amaze me." Out of this discovery Dr. Wilson has become internationally known for his therapy of "Christianity in Medicine." No matter the nature of your stress, prayer changes things. Dr. Joseph Daniels, noted New York psychiatrist, agrees.

Whether your problems are in the home, in the office, at school or on the job, the bottom line is the same. For example, many of our friends know acute financial stress these days. If you have money problems, look at Malachi 3:7–12 and Isaiah 58:6–8 and chapter 61. If you return all your tithes as property of God's— not yours—and do your best to take care of your neighbor, you need never worry; God will take care of you! We have never known of a faithful tither who died from hunger.

Self vs. The Golden Rule

The ultimate test which God levies on you is the same as the Savior lived Himself: *Compassion*. This is the perfect measure of self-worth against the ego of self-esteem and the narcissism which says, "I before you, and you after me."

"Me first" is the infant's cry. Self-preservation is the animal's instinct. In human adults it is a sure road to stress. Whether in finances or diet or sex, the other way is best. The husband who protects his wife in tender patriarchal style, will make no demands of her that he would not make if he were in her place. The loving wife serves her husband and family as unto God.

The Golden Rule does not say that I should argue with my wife if she appears in an argumentative mood. What it does say is that we should settle matters before we go to bed that night.[12] Truly, those couples who practice this principle of settling disagreements or quarrels daily never have to face the divorce court. And the families who pray together morning and evening *in a loving and sharing way* will together see eternal day.

The Golden Rule is for children, too. The Fifth Commandment specifies that they should always be thoughtful of their parents. Many parents, especially mothers, are daily drained from picking up after their children and husbands, when the youngsters and husbands should be picking up after themselves! Children can start to work when they start to walk. They can learn to put things away as well as to get them out. We have spoken and written this concept many times, and when it is carefully and consistently practiced early in life, children become delights instead of ogres.

Such personal discipline should always be united with the clasp of God. Your mind plays an important part in overcoming distress and disease. Positive attitudes and emotions and a sound program of exercise produce positive chemical changes in the body developing happy hormones called endorphins which in turn help build nerve force and reduce stress. Endorphins are your body's natural opiates. They work much like any powerful drug. In fact some specialists are of the opinion that the endorphins are hundreds of times more powerful as painkillers even than morphine.

Your Dress and Your Health

For both adults and children, even preschoolers these days, dress is one of the most stressful of problems. It is often the focus of the peer syndrome; this is one reason many parents give for teaching at home. If you are a slave to fashion and your children are beholden to their peers, you will likely have a health battle for the lifetime of your family. Consider several areas which you sooner or later will face, if you are not facing them now:

Body Temperature

To provide proper body warmth means to be warm enough when your environment is cold and cool enough when the climate is warm, you should have cotton-type clothing or other highly absorptive materials next to your body whenever possible. For infants, during warm weather, take care not to handle a hot little body with sweaty, grimy or salty hands. In cold weather you will see that they are well clothed, particularly in the extremities. If their arms and legs become cold, their abdominal organs tend to become congested; this is especially true if you have tight bands around their thighs or tummies, and is an almost sure guarantee of colic.

This is part of the lesson I learned from Dr. Erwin Syphers in Tokyo, as we mention in Chapter 12 [Liquids]. If you want to be sure that you have healthy lungs and digestive system, be sure that your blood is flowing freely from your heart to all your extremities. However, if your hands, feet, arms, and legs are cold, your blood vessels will be constricted, restricting the flow of blood. This slowed circulation is one of the surest ways to become congested inside your lungs and abdominal area. Dr. Syphers told me to put on some long underwear and do it quickly. I did and, along with my free use of water, I received healing of a serious bronchial ailment that had been with me for too many months.

Style

You may not always feel stylish, although with some planning even that problem can be solved to a reasonable degree. But you will have to make up your mind whether to choose fashion and stupidity or health and common sense.

Speaking of common sense, some years ago the students in an English class in a large Buffalo, New York, high school told their teacher they were disgusted with the trends in student garb: boys in tight jeans or shorts, no sox, shirts with tails flapping out; and girls with tight skirts or shorts, blouses without bras or other underclothing, ad infinitum.

Out of their discussion came a plan they called "Buffalo's Magic Mirror." They installed large mirrors at the head of each stairway as a personal check on how one looked. And what did they prescribe? The boys had to wear sox, tucked-in shirts, properly fitted trousers, and even ties and jackets or sweaters. Girls had to wear similarly fitting clothes which exuded modesty and wholesomeness. To the delight and astonishment of students and teachers alike, the dress code changed the behavior of the entire high school.

There is actually a close relationship not only between clothes and stress, but also between clothes and food. If you want to keep cool in the summer, you should not only wear loose fitting materials, preferably of cotton, but also eat lighter foods, particularly emphasizing fruits and vegetables. Exclude heavy or sweet or fatty or high protein foods. Finally drink plenty of *water,* and drink it in between meals!

Color, Cover and Cost

Light clothing colors reflect the sun instead of absorbing it as dark things do. Long sleeves are also much more healthful than most of us realize. The stress of chilling in winter and the sensation of extreme overheating in exposure to summer sun often adversely affects our adrenals—our temperature meters—and brings stress on our nervous system.

And clothing another extremity is also helpful: the head. A light hat in midday sun will help to keep your head cool. And a warm headdress in winter will keep much of your body heat from escaping this extremity.

Perhaps you have already found that you should not go shopping when a new style comes in, but should shop for quality. A few dollars more for good materials usually pays off well in the long run. Both Dorothy and I found that such quality clothes do not have to be cleaned or pressed as often, are less likely to rip at the seams, last *a lot* longer, and simply look better. If you have to budget, as we have always done, save your money, mending as necessary until sales come on which offer high quality for low prices. There is a lot of education here, valuable lessons to pass on to your children in frugality, judgment, and enterprise. Many of our friends (like us) have not been above purchasing items at used clothing boutiques like, say, the Salvation Army or Goodwill where sometimes you can find a $20 tie or shirt or swim trunks for a dollar.

And all of us should take care to clothe our feet properly. If the weather is very cold, your feet, like the rest of your body, are better clothed with several layers of sox than one thick layer. And shoes should fit comfortably, with good support, and heels that are reasonably flat.

Healthy Feet and Stress

I remember well as a teenager having trouble with my feet. I thought my problem was with shoes that were not wide enough until a perceptive shoe store clerk prescribed shoes a size longer. I have never had trouble since. It is sad that out of ignorance or vanity so many, especially women, cripple their feet, and then pay a dear price after the feet are deformed, never to walk in comfort again. This directly distresses one's health unless some skilled surgeon or podiatrist can (expensively) correct the problem created by poorly fitted footwear.

Mind Over Body

Dorothy has a little prayer plaque near her desk which she feels has been helpful to her as she pleads for "the serenity to accept the things" she cannot change, gains "courage to change" the things she can and receives the "wisdom to know the difference." Norman Cousins has told me of his experience of overcoming pain by use of mind over matter. But when that mind is combined with the Mind of God, no power can excel it.

And your *attitude* will help! Colonel Charles "Chuck" Mayo (who was an office mate for a while in Manila) often declared that at least 80 percent to 90 percent of all *physical* illness at his famed Mayo Clinic "originated in the mind." Dr. Wilson is even more specific. He suggests a firm 90 percent, from his experience as a Christian psychiatrist.

Psychosomatic (mind-body) relationship is often illustrated by the use of placebos. We have a dear friend who has been taking heavy doses of pain-killing drugs for a severe pelvic injury. A quiet Christian nurse tried a combination of placebo and prayer, and soon the patient was injecting himself with sterile water and developing strength without knowing that he wasn't taking drugs. It should be remembered, however, that such addiction is not to be trifled with, for most addicts get so used to the mechanics of the "fix" that they think they "can't stand it" if they don't have that needle.

Unnecessary Fears

Dr. Warren Peters, a vascular surgeon turned health educator, shows how stress begets cancer and warns against unnecessary fears.[13] He reminds us that "Perfect love casts out fear."[14] One of the most dramatic examples of need for such love is the divided family: Cancer is significantly more common among divorced adults than married people.[15] Among people widowed before age 35, cancer afflicts ten times as many as it does the unwidowed.[16]

Your mind does markedly influence your immune system, also. Your body is best defended by a happy mind. "Helplessness and loneliness may be two of the strongest stressors that are known to the human being."[17] And guilt can be likened to loneliness as made so clear in Psalm 38. Often this "is sublimated into alcoholism or obesity."[18] Surely a merry heart does good like a medicine. You will be given perfect peace when your mind is stayed on God.

If we will treat our children as we treat our favorite pets, or as any animal mother will treat her young, and let them grow up naturally with our firm and loving guidance, we will effectively remove much of the stress in young lives. If we do not pressure our children to open up from the outside, God will open them up from the inside just like He makes a rosebud bloom. For more information on children and stress, see Chapter 19 on "Rearing Healthy Children."

Guilt and Stress

Finally, there is *guilt*—the stress which lingers with most of us more than any other. Why, we wonder, did we act impatiently to our spouse or our children that morning when they had only been trying to help? Why didn't we help that family in need who had to leave town? Why did we have improper feelings toward another woman or man? We must do two basic things:

First, we must ask God through Christ to help us to surrender fully to Him, so that our hearts become selfless and we pass on the grace of Christ to others instead of indicting them. This will bring us patience and compassion and forgiveness in love as we come to know God better. For to know God is to love Him, the Source of all love. We will be like Him, for we shall see Him as He is. And guilt will disappear like the smog in a west wind.

Second, we must set out to love our enemies. It may be that we cannot change them, but this admonition in Matthew 5:44 will surely change us! This is the greatest test of character we know, the surest test of our Christianity if we are Christians—or of our principles, if we are not! To love our enemies, we must forgive them. This is God's condition for His forgiveness.[19] If there is a problem we need to settle with them, the remedy is offered in Matthew 18:15–17.

Another admonition: in these days of rampant court suits, avoid them whenever possible; such actions nearly always create more stress. The Christian Legal Society, which any Christian lawyer will know, offers arbitration in cases which normally would be taken to court, and for very little cost.

Using Common Sense

Even as you read this book, remember this: We do not urge extremes or rigidity in diet and general lifestyle. And stress comes in a thousand ways, from computers with their visual and coordinative syndromes to the neighbor's unfriendly dog (he relieves stress if he is friendly). We simply offer a smorgasboard of proven methods in most areas of our lives. Select from them as God gives you wisdom and courage to change. If you wanted to restore a Rolls Royce, you couldn't do better than to take it to the maker. We do not say that if you do not do everything we suggest, you will be wheeled to the hospital or early to the grave. We prefer that you make your own assessments, but do it with knowledge and certainty that the Creator has a design. Try, like Dr. Wilson, to surrender all to the Hands of God, to trust Him as *your* Maker.

. . . your children . . . bring them up
in the nurture and admonition of the
Lord.

Ephesians 6:4

19

Rearing Healthy Children

After we began writing this chapter—sort of writing from back
to front—we had coincidental experiences by mail and phone. Our
friend Dan Matthews wanted us to meet Lee Stanley of the Wings
Foundation of Agoura, California. And Tami Romani called us in
behalf of Bobbi Valentine and Dr. James Dobson to arrange another
series of "Focus on the Family" broadcasts. Our visit with Lee
and Linda Stanley showed us how Wings was matching juvenile
convicts with mature Christian "big brothers"—and rehabilitating
87 percent of these youngsters by introducing them to Jesus.

In the concurrent mail came a then confidential letter from Dr.
Dobson, a member of a Presidential commission, graphically describing the depredations of pornography. The central concern of
both these men was the ignorance, indifference or evil example
of parents to their own children. We believe that it is crucial in a
book like this to alert you to potential emotional and physical health
problems of children.

All the principles given in other chapters are applicable to children,
but a few special cautions are given here to alert you to proven
methods of preventing health problems which seem to be developing
early in life on the American lifestyle. The health of your children
will be largely determined by both parents' lifestyles during preg-

nancy and early months after birth. More detail on starting out right is laid down succinctly in our book, *Home Grown Kids.*

The Jewels: Consistency and Self-Discipline

Also remember that in this time of societal turmoil and stress, your children need all the stability they can get. Their feelings of security are absolutely dependent on your consistency, love, and firmness as well as regularity and routine. In turn this will reduce stress on both you and your children.

Family health involves the mind as well as the body. It depends on the will and good judgment as well as nutrition, exercise, and breathing. We remind you that we speak of discipline as *control,* not punishment, and self-discipline as *self-control,* not masochism. Such control must start at birth and be carried out consistently throughout your children's lives or disaster will befall you. Your goal for your youngsters of eventual worthy self-discipline will be reached as you gradually build their ability to control themselves and concurrently release your parental control. This subject is treated thoroughly in our forthcoming book on creative discipline.

Eating Habits

Specialists on children's eating problems will usually tell you that there are no problem children, only problem parents! Babies arrive in this world without any habits and also without the ability to reason and judge. They don't even have any food prejudices. Their eating patterns are basically *learned by your example, manner, and training.*

Repeated actions form habits, and habits in their turn form character to last for time and eternity. You as parents have the responsibility to train these habits "in the way they should go." Often it takes only two or three repeated acts to lock in a habit, and children being naturally sinful (like you and I), will often lean more to evil ways than good. So you must use divinely endowed wisdom, firmness, self-control, and common sense along with an abundance of love to act in the baby's stead until he is able to control himself.

You can train your baby's appetite to "eat to live or to live to eat," by the way you respond to his real needs—not simply for self-gratification or as a panacea to fulfill his emotional whims, but "in due season, for health and not for drunkenness." And you will do this on a realistic schedule that fits both his body rhythms and your family program. This will not only enhance his health, but also his disposition, emotional security, and mental efficiency. It will also build his self-discipline.

Many adults fondly wish their mothers had helped them to control their appetites at the start. One of our friends with weight problems told us her mother *never let her get hungry.* She was fed to appease every hurt or imaginary need—essentially one meal a day—*all day.* Both quality and quantity must be sensibly monitored for children, because they do not have ability to choose what is best. Obesity, bulemia, anorexia, and even suicide have many of their roots in childhood. One of the problems, of course, is the taste pattern for sugar, fats, and other empty calories which is often established ignorantly or carelessly.

Using Your Head

Suppose you are serving dessert—apple pie and ice cream. Children normally eat much less of other foods than adults, but pretty well expect to have an equal share in the dessert. Let's say that dad is a man of average weight, 160 pounds—and because he is active he needs 3,000 calories a day. Mother weighs 128 pounds and needs 2,000 calories. But Johnny weighs 40 pounds, and because he is also an active little boy, needs 1500 calories. When each has an equal serving of this dessert of 500 calories, one-third of Johnny's total meal was of empty calories with few minerals and vitamins. And in proportion to his weight, he ate four times as many empty calories as his dad! All of this in a small child whose immunities are not yet well established!

When our daughter, Kathie, was a teenager, she was concerned about gaining too much weight as is so easy during those maturing years. She bought her lunch at the school cafeteria and noted that many of her friends did not eat all of what was on their plate but threw it in the garbage. In her mind, this helped them not to gain unwanted weight; yet she indicated that the wasted food consisted of vegetables, salad, and so on, which she had learned was important for a balanced meal. When Dorothy suggested that she might need to eliminate some higher calorie items even at home and make certain choices which were available at school, she said, "But, Mother, you taught me to like everything!" Indeed, she does, but always keeps her weight under control and now is helping her little ones form good health habits.

We are grateful for the eating style our children have as adults, such as eating breakfast cereal without sugar, but we also wish we had taught them other things we have learned since. So now they are un-learning some not-so-good habits we didn't know about when they were little. Too bad they didn't learn the right way at first and not have to retrain their appetites.

Togetherness at Mealtime

Mealtime should be a happy time for the family—a time for good fellowship and loving relationships between parents and children to establish family roots and to cherish for a lifetime. Lateness or too many absences and early departures from the family table greatly discount the quality of family togetherness and good manners. They should be rare.

Television or radio or newspaper should not be allowed to intrude on developing the almost lost art of conversation at the table or anywhere. Use this opportune time, as Deuteronomy 6:7 (NIV) suggests: "to impress [God's words] on your children [by talking] about them when you sit at home." Don't use the lecture method. Don't often ask questions requiring "yes" or "no" answers. Use *whys* and *hows,* doing a reasonable part of the talking, learning how to question, think, analyze and draw conclusions.

Mealtime Rules

Although table decorum is part of child training, try to avoid controversial subjects at mealtime, as well as formal discipline. *Establish your rules well ahead of time,* and if you are consistent, you can have a peaceful meal.

More often than not when children dillydally, protest or are not interested in eating, parents will coax, cajole, force or bribe with dessert. These must be understood as absolute no-nos. There will be no whining or arguing about food. They can get down from the table if they are not agreeable, and will not starve if they are not allowed to return during that meal.

Problems usually arise from the *size* of servings given to children. *Reasonable, limited* preferences should be respected, but children can be trained to like almost everything that is good for them. Since children's appetites may vary at different times, it is better, for a balanced meal, to dish up *very small portions of everything that is served. The portions should add up to less than you expect them to eat,* with the smallest serving being things they like least. Then allow them to return for second or third helpings. If they tend to be overeaters, they will need to be restrained and retrained.

We repeat, if they do not finish what you have first served, they should be immediately, but pleasantly, excused with the understanding that no food will be available until the next regular meal. In no case should a child be given a handout between meals regardless of begging or tears. It is best to serve them the unfinished food at the next meal in the same state in which they left it. If you are calm and consistent, this will be an accepted procedure and will not need to be repeated.

If illness is the reason for loss of appetite, the skipped meal may be the best possible medicine. And if you have been kind and pleasant about the whole operation, you will not have a guilty conscience for being "hard on them." Even two or three missed meals will not harm children if they have adequate water to drink. When they are hungry, they will enjoy the food that is set before them.

The Fussy Eater

In some extreme cases, total retraining is necessary. First, *totally* eliminate between-meal snacks—juice, fruit, or any morsel of anything—so that your children will be hungry *every* meal. You may be surprised to learn that most children do much better on only two meals a day—breakfast as early as needed and dinner five or six hours later, sometimes with a piece of fresh fruit two or three hours before bedtime.

Any food that tends to be disliked should be introduced by itself in small quantities at the beginning of the meal. If it is eaten without any fussing or arguing, other acceptable, and even favorite, healthful foods (not junk foods or desserts) should follow. This food should be consistently used *every* meal—morning, noon or night—until accepted willingly and should be included second in order with the next food introduced, so it won't be forgotten.

If there is any fussing or whining, excuse your children promptly and proceed as stated above. Strong-willed children may hold out a long time, but if you give in even once, it will be harder the next time and eventually they may have to pay the price with poor health. It is a law of the mind that if there is any hope of your weakening, your children will persist, but if they see there is no possibility of getting their way, they will accept the inevitable and make their adjustments.

Other less drastic devices may help with an ordinary fussy eater. For example, you can involve your children in cooking, beginning with foods they like. Also, children who have problems with such things as cooked peas, carrots, asparagus or even broccoli may be more willing to eat them as raw finger foods. Try peeling the large stems of broccoli and see how tender and sweet the inside is. There is no virtue in making sauces, casseroles or other mixed foods if they are disliked. Some children prefer each food by itself and this is probably a reasonable request.

Sleeping Problems

Eda LeShan comments[1] about the virtual epidemic of sleeping problems in recent years. She is evidently old enough to remember thirty years ago when she was a nursery school teacher and such problems were relatively rare. She attributes this problem to current lifestyle pressure with its superbaby preoccupation, including early schooling, mothers in the work force with limitation of love and attention, late bedtimes, food additives, television, and so on.

She recommends, as do we, "a routine they can count on." They need to know what to expect, and this brings security. Calm, soothing days and a ritualistic, regular, and consistent bedtime will make life a lot healthier and happier for you and them, especially when you provide such quieting activities as a warm bath, a childlike story, and prayer.

Building Sound Habits

Habits take a firm hold early in life. We watched a young couple struggle to get their little one to take a nap when they were attending a series of meetings for the day. The baby had become accustomed to a semi-darkened room, quiet music, and a rocking chair each afternoon at nap time. When all these conditions were not available, both the baby and the parents were frustrated. This loving mother had in a sense locked herself and her child into constraints which were more a hindrance than a help.

Music, quiet, and semi-darkness are all good in their place, but we reaped many benefits from teaching our children to sleep wherever and whenever it was necessary. Traveling, necessary in our work, made such adaptability vital to the happiness of all of us. Whether in someone's home, in our car or in a hotel, our children learned that when they were put to bed, they were to go to sleep. It had so long been an accepted part of their lifestyle that there was never any question.

Babies and Sleep

Yale physician T. Berry Brazelton says that sleep problems are probably the issue parents consult him about most. They even ask him for drugs "until the child gets into the habit." Since there is no such drug, he feels that parents should *teach* children to sleep but it takes some practice and determination.[2] Whether good or bad, a child becomes locked into whatever habits you allow him to form.

Babies do not know night from day when they are born. Even though most of them eventually learn to sleep through the night, we have helped some parents at their wit's end whose little ones were still disturbing them several times a night when they were sixteen months and older. This is hard on one's health and marriage! Training, of course, can begin any time, but the trauma for both child and parent is much greater as he grows older, for the child's will becomes stronger and more resistant—his crying much more insistent and persistent.

Most parents succeed in such training best from day one, even in the hospital, because *sleeping and eating patterns are formed from birth*. We are speaking here, of course, of a normal, healthy, full-term baby. *Though strictly an option*, and fully by their choice, parents who have had the loving firmness to follow these few suggestions have come back to thank us for the rest it has brought them to cope with other children and/or the cares of the day. This is not parental indifference, but the deepest kind of love—which understands the damage indulgence can wreak.

A little extra loving attention for play, or even fussing toward the end of the day, can help to make your baby tired enough to sleep through one or more middle-of-the-night feedings, giving you at least six—and preferably eight—hours of uninterrupted sleep. Feed your child *regularly* during the day and be sure he has been offered water between feedings so that he will not be very hungry or thirsty. You will find more *hows* and *whys* on this in our book, *Home Grown Kids*, in *Better Late Than Early* and our book on discipline from the developmental point of view (due in 1987).

Since the sleep cycle for newborns, begun in the womb, follows a rhythm of about three hours during the night, he will likely squirm, make little noises, whimper or even cry at the end of each of these sleep cycles. At this point, by leaving him alone in the dark and quiet, as long as he is not ill, you are encouraging him to maintain a somewhat semi-awake period instead of an alert state and he will soon drift back to sleep. You can start with one omission of feeding and later stretch this out to a full night's sleep for you and the baby.

Our children were each close to eight pounds in birth weight so Dorothy decided to put them on a four-hour schedule, breast-fed, of course. They were both trained to sleep through the night from birth, so this meant nearly eight hours of uninterrupted sleep for us. We feel that the four-hour interval between feedings was good for their digestion also, since they were less likely to spit up *because they were not too full*. They gained well enough for Dennis to outgrow me in height, and for Kathie to outgrow Dorothy.

Of course, if your babies are ill or if they have any other problem, your techniques may need to be altered to suit the situation. Yet, in general, too quick a response to a call or cry may make you a slave to their whims. If you are sold on the family bed, that is also your option, but you should study carefully to determine if it is a lifestyle both you and your spouse can justify and accept over the long run. Whether or not such a practice encourages good sleep patterns apparently has not been established as far as we know, yet such patterns should be our overriding goal.

Spitting Up

The use of infant seats in which babies recline at a 60 degree angle has been found to cause backflow of the contents of the stomach into the esophagus after eating. The result is internal burning (or heartburn) because of the acidity of the reflux. Though more severe disorders could be the actual cause, our suggestion is to lay your baby on his tummy and dispense with the infant seat.[3]

Care of the Teeth

Dental health specialists are saying that parents should cleanse their babies' gums with small pieces of clean gauze wrapped around their finger even before their first teeth appear. These primary teeth need care to prepare for the permanent teeth, not only to save space in the jaw for the permanent teeth, but to assure good eating habits and the proper development of the jaw and face. Brushing to remove bacterial plaque can begin by the age of two to three with close supervision to assure thoroughness. And remember that putting your children to bed with bottles of anything other than water, even fruit juice, makes their teeth vulnerable to decay.

Lifestyle Effects on Sexual Development

Early sexual maturity is thought to be caused primarily from chemical additives in meat—given to the animal to induce rapid development. It is called "precocious puberty syndrome" and includes early enlargement of breasts and early menstruation in girls—a signal of the menarche or ability to reproduce—and enlarged testicles in boys, and growth of pubic hair and acne in both. Flesh foods are among the leading causes here. Drugs or hormones for promoting growth, antibiotics and herbicides are suspect, but the government's monitoring program does not seem to keep these potentially dangerous substances off the market.[4]

And that is not all. Even without chemical additives, diets high in animal fat encourage the growth of hormone-producing bacteria and particularly affect the levels of prolactin, estrogen, and testosterone. The resulting changes are noticeable in the onset of maturity in young women. Girls on low-fat diets begin menstruating at about age sixteen while those on high-fat diets begin as early as eleven or twelve.

These early maturing girls are also likely to have their periods farther apart, with longer, heavier flow and more pain if a high-fat diet is continued. Menopause—the cessation of menstruation—

will take place *later* on high-fat diets—closer to fifty years rather than forty-six—the average age for women on low-fat programs. The same hormones from animal food are also suspect in contributing to breast cancer. Similar, though not so obvious, are the effects on men. Parents should contemplate the possible effects on children of this abnormally early sexual development.

Aspirin Debate

Though some studies have suggested that children given aspirin for either the flu or chicken pox were more likely to develop Reye's syndrome than children who didn't get aspirin, other experts expressed reservations about the studies. In any case, many health officials and pediatricians are advising parents not to use aspirin during these viral illnesses.[5]

Vocal Problems

Encourage your children to speak and play in well-modulated tones. We do not suggest that they should never be allowed to yell, but raunchy yelling and screaming as a general pattern can cripple their vocal chords for life, often inducing growths in their throats.

Stress in Young Children

Whether you are a parent or grandparent, you should be aware that the increase in stress-related problems in children is phenomenal. Symptoms are school phobia, eating disturbances, depression, aggression, and, eventually, at the teen-age level, suicide. Along with the superbaby syndrome which involves parental pride taking precedence over the good of the child, one of the biggest reasons for this stress is the early institutionalizing of little children—putting them in school before they are ready.

Extensive research on the developmental needs of young children by analysis of more than 8,000 studies, besides specific studies at Stanford University, University of Colorado Medical School, and Andrews University, strongly indicates that the young child is not mature enough to handle Day Care, Preschool, Kindergarten or even the Primary grades before he is in the range of eight to ten years old and preferably later. Before that, he does not have the capability to cope with the separation from you, exposure to large groups, conflicting moral standards, peer pressure and competition, and pressure to achieve in areas in which he is unready.

Such institutionalization, especially when it is not urgently necessary, perhaps amounts to the most pervasive form of child abuse and neglect today. This is verified by specialists and scholars ranging from Dr. Martin Engel, then Director of the National Demonstration Center in Early Childhood Education,[6] to Dr. John Bowlby, London psychiatrist who heads the children's division of the World Health Organization.[7]

Dr. Engel insists that no matter how we rationalize our purpose in putting our children early into any out-of-home care, they usually feel rejected. Dr. Bowlby considers this more harmful to the child than being mistreated by an alcoholic father. And Cornell's Urie Bronfenbrenner points out that the devastation of peer dependence and its loss of family values is more the fault of the rejecting parent than the rejected child.[8]

Because of their special endowment of intelligence, very bright children are unusually vulnerable to stress. Several typical characteristics may contribute to their high risk: (1) their perfectionist tendencies, (2) the difference between their emotional-social development and their mental development, (3) their supersensitivity to adult problems, (4) and their possible boredom when exposed to the same process used for the average child in the classroom, yet sensitivity to yours or their teacher's excessive achievement demands. For more on early schooling, see *Home Grown Kids*.

Heart Disease Ahead

American children of school age have been found to average above 180 milligrams of cholesterol per 100 cc. of blood which is 60 to 80 points higher than the ideal. According to the American Health Foundation, a non-profit research group working on preventive medicine, these children may be headed for heart disease. They declare that this is largely caused by excess fat in the diet, particularly whole-fat dairy products and red meats.

The Reader's Digest of March, 1986 ("The Dismal Truth About Teen-Age Health," pages 103 to 107), reports that teenagers have significantly higher blood pressure than they did in the 1960s. Some

98 percent of 360 children, ages 7 to 12 had at least one risk factor for heart disease; more than half had three or more risk factors, increasing as grade levels increase. Too much salt and fat were given as the cause. They also have a significantly higher percentage of body fat than their counterparts 20 years ago. When the American hot dog contains 89 percent fat, with a rough equivalent in cheeseburgers, is it any wonder?

Physical Unfitness

When the Presidential Physical Fitness Award of 85-percent performance level in six tests, from sit-ups to the 50-yard dash was given in 1976, 15 percent of high-school students qualified. In 1983 the same test was given to 84,000 students and less than one percent of those tested reached this level.

Both gym and health classes have not only declined in number and quality in schools, but now children do less walking and biking to school. When you add their average six hours daily watching TV, such deterioration in fitness development is understandable. The lesson is clear and it is up to you to decide what you are going to do about your children.

Sleep Deficit

The report is not much more encouraging about other factors of teen-age health. Going to the bedroom or to bed at night does not necessarily mean that your children are going to sleep. Earphone music with no relation to lullabies, TV sets in the bedroom, and other distractions cause young people to be deficient in sleep when their actual need, according to a Stanford University Sleep Research Center study, is about nine hours a night.

The report concludes that as a consequence of these three areas of declining health, the mental health of teen-agers is in serious jeopardy. And conspicuous by its absence is positive parental time and attention. In 1979 the death rate for 15- to 24-year-olds was the only age category higher than it had been 20 years ago. The suicide rate had tripled since 1976. Many things need to be done to help turn this disastrous picture around, but we agree with one commentator that "Parents are the key in addressing the problem." Television should never be available in your children's rooms, and preferably no radio. It should be a quiet place at bedtime.

You made all the delicate inner parts
of my body, and knit them together in
my mother's womb.

Psalm 139:13, 14 NIV

20

When Families Are Pregnant

When Dorothy was pregnant with Dennis, our first child, I am certain that I suffered more from concern and curiosity than she. I am not by nature a worrier, and I wasn't supposed to be bothered by her female problems. Yet, caught as I was in the New Guinea jungles during World War II, her happiness, safety, and the prospects of our firstborn-to-be made me an explicit participant in her pregnancy even though she was a vast ocean away.

Father's in There, Too

I had heard that prospective fathers generally gave little attention to the whole creative process of making a new human being, and wondered if I were unusual. After talking with dads who have much more experience than I, there is no doubt in *my* mind now that fathers who love their families do get involved. Witness the thousands of dads-to-be who happily share pregnancies with their wives via the Bradley, Lamaze, and Leboyer plans and who eventually "coach" their precious women through childbirth. And indeed they do become more precious in this sharing.

Perhaps just as important is the planning well before pregnancy! Habits, attitudes, and health of both parents can be crucial to the birth of a healthy normal child. Medical science still knows little about the causes of many abnormalities and handicapped children, but it knows enough to be certain that you cannot be too careful. You may not be able to control all the outcomes, but you can be in there doing your best. Our book, *Home Grown Kids,* may help you look ahead, understand how your children develop, how to care for them during and after pregnancy, and how to have real fun being parents.

Such a spirit is much more prevalent today than it was a half a century ago, or even ten years back. Gallup Polls estimate that as many as 80 percent of the fathers today are present at their children's birth. A similar number change diapers and at least two out of every five fathers bathe their new offspring. So this chapter is for both mothers and dads, and even for older children.

Physical Conditioning

Basic nutrition and general physical fitness not only help to produce a healthy baby, but will make the birth itself much easier. Remember the situation among the Hebrew women when Moses was born. Pharaoh had ordered the Hebrew midwives to kill all the boys as soon as they were born, so as to cut down the population explosion. From Pharaoh's point of view, the midwives were not cooperative, and he rebuked them for letting the baby boys live. But he obviously accepted their explanation that "the Hebrew women have their babies so quickly that we can't get there in time! They are not slow like the Egyptian women!" (Exodus 1:19, LB)

The fact is that *toil in the open air* required of the Hebrew slaves caused them to be in good physical condition and childbirth was comparatively easy while Egyptian women were sedentary. Even now Arabic women, who are racially related to the Hebrews and lead physically strenuous lives, require little assistance in childbirth. Considering the large population of Hebrews, midwife services were evidently not in much demand since only two are named! (See Exodus 1:15.)

There probably is no area of health that cherishes more *old wives' tales* than pregnancy. They tell about diet, weight, rest, exercise, tastes, comforts, and dangers. Let's examine a few of these taboos, and try to find answers that make sense. We believe that we should keep pregnancy in perspective and not flail wildly at prospective mothers who are struggling to keep their wits.

TALE #1, SALT

Use very little salt, lest you retain fluids. Some physicians once believed that using less salt would avoid toxemia. Unless you have hypertension, or tend to be intemperate in the use of salt, it is no longer *sharply* restricted. Just be aware that salt is already prominently seasoned into most processed foods, not to mention such obvious items as salted crackers, pretzels, and chips. Even though your body does tend to lose more salt than normal during pregnancy, most everyone overdoes salt anyway, so just take care. And physicians do advise that iodized salt be used. See Chapter 9, "Spice and Everything 'Nice,' " for more on the use of salt.

TALE #2, SWEETENERS

If you are pregnant, you should not use sugar substitutes. There is no evidence to date that aspartame, saccharin, and their namesakes such as Nutrasweet and Equal are any more detrimental to pregnant women than anyone else. We naturally would prefer to see less of these unnatural sweeteners used, and our tastes adjusted to more natural foods, yet to single out such women is not appropriate, except 1) for those who may have metabolic problems which preclude these sweeteners, and 2) for women who have a desire to give their offspring the best of nutrition and who realize that the more natural and wholesome their food, the better the health is likely to be of the little one inside them.

If you insist on sweets, let them be in or with foods which provide adequate vitamins and minerals for sound digestion, such as whole wheat crackers and 100 percent whole wheat or mixed-grain breads instead of white. If there is any doubt, the advice of an experienced physician or nutritionist should be sought.

TALE #3, OVEREATING

Since she must eat enough for two, and your little one has to grow almost from nothing, she should eat twice as much. This does seem likely because of her heavy needs for iron, calcium, folic acid, and other vitamins and minerals. Yet for the first three months of pregnancy, the mother-to-be actually needs only about 150 more calories each day or about 15 percent more than normal.

For the remainder of her pregnancy her energy requirement moves up to about 350 additional calories daily—an amount which can be met normally by an extra sandwich or helping of entrée. What she *must* be careful about is the *selection* of her food so that it meets her larger requirements for vitamins, minerals, and other nutritive needs.[1]

TALE #4, WEIGHT CONTROL

You should not allow your weight to increase more than several pounds beyond the extra weight of the baby you are carrying. This idea has several origins: 1) the fear that you "will get in the habit" of being fat, 2) that you will lose your figure permanently, and 3) you will have a smaller baby with a probably easier delivery. There is more truth in the first two than in the third. Depending on the woman's normal frame, from 20 to 30 pounds of added weight is not considered out of line by leading obstetricians—who believe that it is justified by extra fluids, placenta, breast weight, and reserves for breast feeding.

Weight should be added gradually over the period of pregnancy, with most of it after the first three months. If she experiences a sudden sharp gain, she should promptly consult her physician. Her mate would do well to realize that she will normally have "crazy" tastes, and may have a tendency to get fat. At this special time she will also need unusual self-control. He can be a bright light in encouraging her to "be beautiful" and not to worry that she won't regain "her old figure." Then, after their baby is born, he should work patiently and wisely with her to help her gradually but surely to regain her firm, normal shape.

TALE #5, PRENATAL DIET

You don't have to worry about what you eat until you are pregnant. The earlier that women can embark on a sound program of nutrition, the better, even from girlhood. The baby will be what the mother is, and to a great extent, what she has been. This is also true of smoking, drugs, and alcohol, and even such simple things as aspirin. These chemicals seem to focus on the tiny little one inside her and are often concentrated several times as much as in the mother.

Mothers who have indulged during pregnancy will find that their newborns will have to go through the agonies of withdrawal that they themselves would have to experience if they were to quit their narcotic habits. A pregnant woman can drink no alcoholic beverages of any kind in any amount without risking her baby's lowered birth weight and prematurity, with even greater possibilities of abnormality, retardation, and so on, if she drinks regularly and substantially.

TALE #6, CRAVINGS

The foods which you normally crave will generally be good for you. Not true, no matter how sound her normal diet may be and how much she knows about nutrition. The principles above should guide. This is perhaps the most important single period of her life to be careful in the selection of her food. And here again her husband can be a gentle strength. This also applies to foods which she may turn against, yet need.

Vitamin B6

A few other bits of information will be helpful to most families anticipating a new arrival. Since morning sickness during at least six weeks near the beginning of the pregnancy is thought to be caused from a lack of Vitamin B6, you may want to concentrate on foods that are rich in this valuable nutrient in order to avoid or reduce such difficulty. B6 is the vitamin that has not been taken out of whole wheat flour and not put back in to "enrich" it. Obviously then, whole wheat products will contain it, as do leafy green vegetables, legumes, bananas, and other whole grains. It is essential to central nervous system function; fat, carbohydrate, and protein metabolism; formation of antibodies; and it maintains sodium/potassium balance as well as helps in this problem.

Drinks

Since caffeine in coffee and tea seriously interfere with iron absorption, so crucial to good blood, these drinks are obviously not desirable for you if you want the best for your baby.

Though cocoa varies in the amount of caffeine it contains, depending on its source, at worst it contains less caffeine than coffee or tea. One of its greatest disadvantages again is the sugar its normal use demands.

We should note that not only is the caffeine in coffee objectionable, but also that it contains many "volatile" or irritant oils. So, whether pregnant or not, male or female, you may find your physician cautious about permitting you even caffeine-free coffees if you have stomach ulcers or other problems of the digestive tract. For more on coffee, tea and cola drinks, see Chapter 12 [Liquids, Inside and Out].

Milk and Allergies

Another caution in the prospective mother's diet is the matter of drinking cow's milk with the possibility of causing allergies in the unborn child. This is addressed in Chapter 7 on Milk, under *Dairy Products*. Other factors about the use of milk are described in Chapter 12 on Liquids.

When a family becomes pregnant, then, it should be considered a family affair. Dad and the children should be sympathetic to mother's special needs and tastes. Together they should exercise her—even more carefully and lovingly than they would the family pet! They should serve her as one especially prepared by God to work with Him as He creates a new person.

> . . . fear the Lord and shun evil. This
> will bring health to your body and nour-
> ishment to your bones.
>
> *Proverbs 3:7, 8*

21

The Other Bible Gospel: Health

God told Moses just what Israel was to do and promised that if they would do what he told them, He would "put none of these diseases upon" them which He had brought upon the Egyptians. And He adds that He is indeed "the Lord that healeth thee" (Exodus 15:26). Forty years later at the crossing of the Jordan River they had no feeble or sick people among them (Psalm 105:37). Moses and Israel were, like Daniel and his friends, testing the promises of the Creator Himself for blessings and health in their day-to-day lives.

Although most of us know little of the history of diet, modern health records of orthodox Jews testify to the wisdom of the ceremonial laws God laid down for their health.

But how about the ancient Egyptians? The science of paleopathology reports that they had many of the same diseases as our modern society. We can tell by their art, medical writings, and mummies. Because of their delusions about the state of the dead, they preserved their dead bodies, and now scientists are able to determine what their diseases were.[1]

Lifestyle Change During the Exodus

First the causes: The lifestyle of the Egyptians had largely influenced the Israelites as noted in their responses to a change during the Exodus. God obviously had to teach them many things, including diet. First, we know that they complained about their vegetarian diet and wailed for the "flesh pots" of Egypt.[2] They also highly valued milk, cheese, and butter.[3]

Archeological evidence shows that olive oil was purchased by Egypt in large quantities from Crete, that they ate the fat and blood of animals (even the modern day Egyptian's favorite sandwich is the fat of meat on white bread), they had ways of refining flour, and stills for brewing beer. Because of their slaves and chariots, the leaders and the well-to-do lived luxurious, sedentary lives. Leaving the table to vomit so as to return to the table to indulge in more food was also a common custom, as it was in Rome. Today we call it "bulemia."

Now the problems: Mummies show evidence of extensive arteriosclerosis, dental caries and abscesses, gallstones, obesity, degenerative arthritis, leprosy, tuberculosis, cancer, parasitic infestation, kidney stones, diabetes, and a number of other diseases, even including poliomyelitis.[4]

So, whether we look at the Scriptures or at archeology's witness, it is clear that God had a wise plan. Man had an appetite and a choice in Eden. He had a chance again before the Great Flood when God predicted a 100 percent chance of rain. He has the same chance today. When he chooses against divinity, he chooses against life, because God is the Source of all life. When he prefers the pathway to death, he is bound to suffer. The questions for you and me, then, are "How good are we at choosing?" and "How skilled are we at changing our habits?"

Firmness in the Right

Dwight Eisenhower changed instantly when he learned that he must give up smoking if he wanted to live. Eisenhower's physician, heart specialist Paul Dudley White, told me that the President's motivation was so strong that he quit that very day. Many men and women, however, will not change even if it is a matter of life and death. On the other hand if you have been close to those who have had spectacular recoveries from serious problems, you have seen the value of dramatic lifestyle change. And you have probably observed that the highest motivation of all is the sincere desire of the Christian to please God, to obey and to glorify the

One who made him. Then He promises that as we do this we may be "transformed by the renewing" of our minds, so that we *can prove* what is the "perfect will of God."[5]

Paul often reminds us that we "are bought with a price," and we are not our own. This is as much a part of the gospel as Christ's death and resurrection, for *our* living sacrifice is our best response to *His* living and dying sacrifice. This means that we will take the best possible care of ourselves so that in every phase of our lives, we will live to glorify God.

When God created man in His own image[6] he was perfect, but when he fell into sin, man began to deteriorate physically, mentally, and morally. Fortunately, God had a plan to redeem man and bring him back to the perfection in which he was created—to restore him to His own image in every way. Those who determine to belong completely to Him do not consider God's plan for their lives merely as a duty, but *love* to glorify Him in every use of their physical, mental, and moral powers.

That Other Law

There is another law, of course, which takes over if we choose not to follow God's way and that is the law of cause and effect. You see it around you—lung cancer from smoking, AIDS from sexual perversion, destroyed minds and bodies from drugs and alcohol, obesity, and distress from overeating and junk feeding. It is spelled out in Galatians 6:7: "Be not deceived; God is not mocked: for whatsoever a man soweth, that shall he also reap."

You will notice that biblical principles of health form the basis for every chapter in this book. Where scientific discoveries conform to these principles, they are applied. Jesus was the way, the *truth* and the life.[7] When science is correctly interpreted, it conforms to Him. He made it!

He always combined His ministry to the soul with ministry to the body and mind. His goal was to make man whole—which is the key to real Christian growth and the challenge of His life to us.[8] Our appetites and passions, as well as our characters themselves, are largely dependent on the health of our bodies.

In-sane! Without Reason

If we knew what was really going on inside our bodies from the way we mistreat them, most of us would be scared. Some of us might even faint. That is precisely what happened recently to a young man who, after offering his girl friend alcohol on top of her normal medication, suddenly sensed that he had risked her life. With little thought of their potential, we regularly introduce into our bodies substances that would horrify us if a friend suggested we give them to our favorite pets: poisons, drugs, and dangerous germs. *Yet we somehow reason that our bodies will take care of themselves.* Indeed they will—up to a point.

In a word, most of us are *insane* about our bodies—meaning "without reason." Only when our bodies begin to take care of themselves—usually through pain—do we briefly come to our senses. And once relieved of distress, how quickly we then forget! In fact, how little we seriously think about it at all!

It may help you to remember that absence of illness does not necessarily indicate good health. A recent striking example was widely admired actress Donna Reed. In December of 1985 she spoke in sympathy for and on behalf of cancer victims without realizing that she herself had cancer. By mid-January of 1986 she was laid to rest, a victim of the very disease she had spoken against.

Because of its God-given vital force, the body can take considerable misuse. When we were originally created, for example, the protective and elaborate mechanism was set up by God to give the unborn babe in the womb every possible benefit of the doubt nutritionally as it develops.

Another good reason for concern about your health is that the Creator designed your body as the only medium through which your mind and soul are developed for the upbuilding of your character. No wonder that Satan directs his temptations to weaken the physical powers. He tried it unsuccessfully with Christ, and now he is trying it desperately on you and me. There is a physiological basis for this. It is partially explained by the ability of a strong body to create electric currents in the body strong enough to counteract disease and maintain mental health and strength.

Dying Ahead of Time

Sadly, both young and old often do not learn until their dying days that health is a gift of life whose alternative is illness, pain, and death. Dr. Milton G. Crane observes that we are living longer, but are living older, sicker. Health brings happiness or misery exactly to your order. In a remarkable cycle and countercycle, the ways of your body determine the sense of your mind and the turn of your mind dictates directly the welfare of your body. This gives new meaning to the invitation, "Let this mind be in you, which was also in Christ Jesus."[9]

When your body is tired, your mind is dull. When your mind is perplexed or weighted with care, your energy level drops; your coordination and poise are impaired. Then the ultimate threat always waits at the door: Physical and mental lethargy nearly always risk self-control which opens the door to moral failure. On the other hand, proper physical habits promote mental superiority and a greater likelihood of moral purity. This is obvious in the contrasts in achievement, behavior, and control in any classroom where students who eat heavily sugared foods can be compared with those who come to school with healthful lunches.

Said another way, health does not depend upon luck. It comes in obedience to the Creator's unalterable natural laws. Wise physicians, physical educators, and athletes know them well, for on them depend physical strength as well as intellectual power and longevity. Although these laws may not be as dramatic as the operating room or the sports arena, they are as absolute as gravity, genetics, sound, and light.

Self-Mastery

Self-direction—self-control—is the key to success. He who is first master of himself rules men. Yet we cannot be masters or ourselves until and unless we choose One to master us who created us. It makes sense for a Rolls Royce owner to go to a dealer certified by the manufacturer to have his car serviced. We would think him stupid if he took it to the alley garage.

Dorothy and I have learned by hard experience that we should go to the best doctor we can find, and to give better heed to God's plans for us. Whenever the two of us went to have physical examinations, Dorothy's cholesterol was consistently higher than mine, though our diet has been essentially the same. My cholesterol level usually ran from 125 to 130, and hers over 200. One physician suggested the reason might be heredity, which is likely enough. But she finally took the advice of friends and went to Weimar for a lifestyle change.

Your Blood—Your Life

The quality of your blood is a good indicator of your lifestyle. No wonder the Bible refers to it as "the life." You may find it worthwhile to read Deuteronomy 12:23–25 and Leviticus 17:10–14. [See Chapter 8, "Those Vege Nuts" for details on this.] All the food constituents whether used as fuel, tissue builders, or as helpers in the growth, health, and work of the tissues are carried in the bloodstream. This vital fluid also carries away waste to be expelled—such as carbon dioxide from the lungs and nitrogen leftovers from the kidneys, bowels, and skin.

The experiences of other patients at Weimar were even more spectacular. One was a physician suffering from diabetes. He had been taking fifty units of insulin a day to survive. Even worse, he had diabetic neuropathy which caused him to have sharp, stabbing pain in his feet. His neurologist had insisted sadly that it was a condition he was going to have to live with the rest of his days. Yet, in less than a week on the Weimar program with its diet, physical therapy (including fomentations, Russian baths, etc.), the pain in his feet was gone, and before long he was walking several miles a day. He was also down to twelve daily units of insulin a day and expected that with continuation of the program at home he soon would be able to eliminate the insulin entirely. He now proclaims widely that he no longer walks on razor blades, but "on cloud nine."

That ten-day program of returning health and vigor to Dorothy (which she extended to twenty days) was a reminder to her of the *ten-day trial* Daniel and his friends specified to the Babylonian chief official in King Nebuchadnezzar's Court. God added His blessing to their efforts and they were obviously in better health than the other young men who had eaten the King's rich food. It was a simple cause-and-effect matter: You are what you eat and become what you live. And Dorothy was also reminded that they obeyed God because they loved Him, not of works that they could boast.

And what was the secret? Obedience to the simple and natural laws we are telling you about in this book. Ern Baxter (see Chapter 2) now tells his listeners not to wait like he did—and millions are doing today—until you have a problem. Why not prevent it? *We remind you once again that there is no happenstance, no chance, about health. There are gracious rewards for careful care of your*

*body and a penalty for every violation of the laws of life, both
mentally and physically, and they tend to accrue as we grow older.*
So let's look ahead: If we sacrifice present pleasures, we are certain
to reap future benefits!

APPENDIX A

T<small>YPICAL</small> F<small>OOD</small> C<small>AUTIONS FROM THE</small> U.S. F<small>OOD AND</small> D<small>RUG</small> A<small>DMINISTRATION</small>
[As developed by Dario Cappucci, DVM, Ph.D. MPH, of FDA]

1. "Antibiotics-in-feed issue to be submitted to PHS committee," *Food Chemical News*. No. 6, Vol. 28. April 14, 1986.
2. Asner, Marti, "Worms that turn good food into bad," *FDA Consumer*, September 1982, 4.
3. Ballentine, Carol, "For oyster and clam lovers, the water must be clean," *FDA Consumer*, 1985.
4. Ballentine, Carol, "Pollution narrows shellfish harvest," *FDA Consumer*, Vol. 19, No. 1, February 1985, 10.
5. Ballentine, Carol, "Who, why, when and where of food poisons (and what to do about them)," *FDA Consumer*, July/August 1982.
6. *Bureau of Veterinary Medicine*, "Monitoring for residues in food-animals," Revised October 1983.
7. *FDA Consumer Memo*, "Antibiotics and the foods you eat."
8. *FDA Consumer Memo*, "Here are some questions and answers about commonly used meat and food additives."
9. *FDA Consumer*, "Primer on three nutrients," Revised January 1981.
10. Harland, Barbara, and Hecht, Annabel, "Grandma called it roughage," *FDA Consumer*, 1984.
11. Hecht, Annabel, "For fruits and vegetables, Americans favor 'fresh'," *FDA Consumer*, October 1985, 7.

12. Hecht, Annabel, "Lab warns cow: Don't drink your milk," *FDA Consumer*, July/August 1985, 31.

13. *Journal of the American Veterinary Medical Association*, "Antibiotics in animal feed and antibiotic resistance subjects of house hearing," Vol. 186, No. 7., April 1, 1985, 662.

14. Kandra, Karen A., "Sulfonamide residues in bob-veal calves," *JAVMA*, Vol. 187, No. 1, July, 1985, 26.

15. Larkin, Tim, "Food fit for a fido," *FDA Consumer*, June 1983.

16. Lecos, Chris, "A closer look at dairy safety," *FDA Consumer*, April 1986, 14.

17. Lecos, Chris, "Dietary guidelines for no-nonsense advice for healthy eating," *FDA Consumer*, November 1985, 10.

18. Lecos, Chris, "Fish and fowl lure consumers from red meat," *FDA Consumer*, October 1985, 19.

19. Lecos, Chris, "Of microbes and milk: Probing America's worst *salmonella* outbreak," *FDA Consumer*, February 1986, 18.

20. Lecos, Chris, "Milk: Cows produce it; man improves it," *FDA Consumer*, June 1982, 16.

21. Lecos, Chris, "The public health threat of food-bourne diarrheal disease," *FDA Consumer*, Vol. 19, No. 9, November 1985, 19.

22. Lecos, Chris, "Reacting to sulfites," *FDA Consumer*, December 1985/January 1986.

23. Lecos, Chris, "Sweetness minus calories = controversy," *FDA Consumer*, Vol. 19, No. 1, February 1985, 18.

24. Lecos, Chris, "Water, the number one nutrient," *FDA Consumer*, November 1983.

25. Miller, Roger W., "Soft drinks and six-packs quench our national thirst," *FDA Consumer*, October 1985, 23.

26. Miller, Roger W., "America's changing diet," *FDA Consumer*, October 1985, 4.

27. *Nutrition and Your Health*, "Dietary guidelines for Americans," Second Edition, 1985.

28. Rados, Bill, "Eggs and dairy foods: Dietary mainstays in decline," *FDA Consumer*, October 1985, 11.

29. Rados, Bill, "Feeding animals wonder drugs and creating super bugs," *FDA Consumer*, Vol. 19, No. 1, February 1985, 14.

30. *Requirements of laws regulations enforced by the U.S. FDA.*

31. Rodricks, Joseph V., "Hazards from nature: Aflatoxins," *FDA Consumer*, Revised October 1980.

32. Rosenberg, Myron C., "Update on the sulfonamide residue problem," *JAVMA*, Vol. 187., No. 7, October 1, 1985, 704.

33. Settepani, Joseph A., "The hazard of using chloramphenicol in food animals," *JAVMA*, Vol. 184, No. 8, April 15, 1984, 930.

APPENDIX B

SOME SAMPLE RECIPES

Here are a few of Dorothy's favorite recipes along with her counsel in using them. These will get you started and tide you over until you get something more complete. If you enclose a self-addressed envelope with your request to "Recipes," Box 9, Washougal, WA 98671, we will be glad to send you a list of up-to-date cookbooks that incorporate the ideals in this book and will help you more and more to progress into a better way.

In changing over to a more healthful diet, start by adapting some of your familiar recipes and substitute or omit the harmful ingredients. For example, suppose a family favorite is lasagna. Use ripe, black olives in chunks or a vegetarian burger (textured vegetable protein) instead of meat, cook whole wheat pasta and make cheese out of nuts—perhaps not all at the same time. Pizza, many kinds of Mexican foods, and Chinese dishes can be made healthfully by omitting devitalized foods and substituting whole plant foods.

Even in the following recipes, use your own creativity and adjust seasonings, amount of liquid, and so on, to your own tastes or desires. As substitutes for oily dressings and sauces, you will notice the combination of grains and nuts with harmless herbs and other seasonings and much use of a good blender to help you adjust to this new foodstyle. Find a good, flexible rubber spatula to clean out your containers or blender "that nothing be wasted."

MAIN DISHES

Tamale Loaf

1 large onion, chopped	1 c. water
1 large clove garlic, minced	1 t. salt
1 chopped green pepper (optional)	½ t. cumin
3 c. tomatoes, fresh or canned	1 c. yellow cornmeal
2 c. corn, whole or creamed	1 can olives, quartered

Cook first five items in water until tender and bring to a boil. Add salt, cumin, and cornmeal gradually, stirring constantly, and cook over low heat until thick. Then add olives. Other seasonings such as paprika, sweet basil, thyme, oregano, or bay leaf may be added as desired. Bake in casserole for 1 hour at 325 degrees. The loaf will be firmer if made a day ahead, refrigerated, and then baked before serving. It will also freeze well. Serve with tomato sauce, if desired.

Option: Millet may be substituted for the cornmeal, but it needs more liquid and longer cooking either on top of the stove in a double boiler or crockpot, or longer baking in a covered casserole. Instead of corn, you might wish to use ½ cup of cashew nut pieces and substitute green ripe olives for the ripe olives.

Holiday Nut Dressing

2 large onions, chopped	2 t. ea. sage/thyme
3–4 stalks celery including tops and leaves	½ t. ea. salt/rosemary/garlic powder
2 T. chicken-like seasoning	1 t. ea. savory/marjoram
2 c. water, approx.	3 t. dried parsley

Cook all together until vegetables are tender. Toss with fork into 1 loaf (12 cups) of whole wheat bread which has been cubed and oven-toasted lightly. Add 1 cup of coarsely chopped walnuts. Serve with brown gravy. (This used to be the best part of the turkey dinner to us years ago and it is still a favorite main dish any day.)

Savory Pinto Beans or Lentils

2 c. pinto beans or lentils	1 large onion, chopped
5 c. water	1 clove garlic, minced
1 t. salt	1 green pepper, chopped
½ t. ea. savory/cumin	3–4 stalks celery, chopped
1 bay leaf	4 c. canned tomatoes
Optional seasonings such as oregano, thyme, or sweet basil	

Soak beans overnight and cook until tender. (Lentils need not be soaked and cook much more quickly than beans.) Several more cups of boiling water may be needed for the beans during cooking unless pressure cooker is used. A crockpot may be used for overnight, set on medium or high heat.

Whether beans have been soaked overnight or not, you can shorten cooking time by bringing them to a boil, turning off the heat, and letting them soak one hour with the lid on before cooking. Some feel that draining the soaking water and adding new water to beans makes them less gas-forming. Thorough cooking is important also to avoid this problem.

Add other ingredients and cook until beans are very tender, and vegetables are done. Serve in bowls, over waffles or toast for breakfast, rice or baked potatoes for a main dish, or as a base for soup or stew to which other vegetables may be added.

Lentil and Nut Roast

1 ½ c. cooked brown rice *or* dry w.w.
  bread crumbs
1 medium onion, chopped

1 c. nut meal
2 c. cooked lentils
½ t. ea. sage/savory/salt

Combine all ingredients and add vegetable juice or water if too dry. Pour into casserole and bake 45 minutes at 325 degrees. Serve with tomato sauce or gravy.

Bean Burgers

3 c. brown rice
3 c. tender, mashed beans
3 T. minced parsley or chives (opt.)
Salt if needed

½ t. ea. sage/celery salt
1 t. onion powder
⅓ c. w.w. flour

Mix well and shape into burgers. Bake on teflon sheet at 350 degrees for about 25 minutes. Serve with tomato sauce or gravy or in a whole wheat bun with sliced tomato, onion, lettuce and/or "cheese."

Haystacks or Tostados

Toast in the oven until crisp, whole or chip-size pieces of tortillas. Over each tortilla or handful of chips, spread mashed savory pinto beans, cooked without tomatoes or any extra juice. Cover with any combination of shredded lettuce or other greens, diced tomatoes, shredded carrots, chopped onions, and sliced olives. Top with "Cheese," Avocado Salad Dressing, thinned mayonnaise or "Sour Cream."

Holiday Almond Loaf

½ c. soaked garbanzos or soy beans
½ c. water
½ c. almonds
½ c. sunflower or other seeds
1 c. boiling water
1 c. oats
1 chopped onion

1 c. bread crumbs
½ c. chopped celery
½ t. salt

Sage, marjoram, onion and garlic powder, dried parsley to taste. Or Chicken-like seasoning as given below.

Soak beans overnight, drain. Blend with water until thick and creamy. Add almonds and seeds and blend to finely chopped consistency. Combine all in bowl and let stand 10 minutes. Press into teflon or sprayed loaf pan or ring mold. Bake at 350 degrees for 45 minutes to 1 hour. Good sliced or in sand.

GRAVY, SAUCES, DRESSINGS, AND SPREADS

Gravy

1 large onion, chopped
3 c. potato or green bean water
3 T. w.w. flour

1–3 T. (approx.) seasoning—sovex, soy sauce, or vegex

Brown flour in skillet. Blend and bring to a boil while stirring constantly.

Golden Sauce

1 ea. med. cooked potato and carrot
½ t. salt

1 c. water
1 T. lemon juice

Blend until smooth. Heat and serve over such vegetables as cauliflower or broccoli.

"Cheese"

1 c. water
⅓ c. flour
1 t. onion powder
¼ c. food yeast flakes
½ c. pimiento or cooked drained tomatoes & ¼ t. turmeric

⅔ c. cashews or sunflower seeds
2 T. lemon juice
¼ t. garlic powder
1 t. salt

Blend all ingredients together until creamy, *except the flour*. Without the flour it may be used as a spread for bread, sauce for baked macaroni, or dressing on salad or vegetables.

When you stir in the flour, it is ready to use on pizza or baked spaghetti, in Mexican food or in layers of lasagna. For cheese toast spread on slices of bread and bake at 400 F. until browned. If you cook it until thick and refrigerate it in a square container, it may be sliced. Or if it is frozen after cooking, it can be grated while frozen.

"Sour Cream" or Mayonnaise

1 c. water
¼ c. cooked rice (optional)
½ t. salt

½ c. cashews or sunflower seeds
3 T. lemon juice

Boil seeds or nuts in the water for 5 minutes. Blend with other ingredients for 1 full minute. Chill before serving. For Mayonnaise: Add a few dates to hot mixture, triple the rice and add ¼ t. ea. celery salt and garlic and onion powder.

Avocado Salad Dressing, Spread or Dip

1 ripe avocado, peeled and mashed
  or blended with other ingredients.

1–2 T. lemon juice
Diced tomato for guacamole

Sprinkle with salt, garlic powder and onion powder to taste. Add enough water, "milk" or skim milk to thin for consistency needed.

Olive-Nut Spread

1 c. almonds
¼ t. ea. garlic/onion powder

1 c. water, approx.
1 can chopped olives

Blend all except olives until smooth, adjusting consistency with water. Add olives without blending.

Dried Fruit Jam or Spread

Simmer or soak overnight any combination of dried fruit with just enough unsweetened fruit juice or water to cover. Balance sweet fruits such as prunes or dates with peaches or pears to desired sweetness. Blend and store in refrigerator. Keeps at least a week.

Breakfast Dishes

Soy-Oat Waffles

1 c. cooked soy beans
2 ¼ c. water

1 ½ c. rolled oats
½ t. salt

Blend for ½ minute. Let stand to thicken while waffle iron is heating. Blend again and pour about 1 ½ cups of batter into hot nonstick waffle iron. If necessary, spray initially with "Pam" or the like. Bake about 8–10 minutes. Don't peak too soon. (We make quite a few at a time, freeze the extras, and heat as needed in the toaster or oven.)

Variation: Yellow cornmeal or other whole grain flour may be substituted for the soy beans.

Toppings: Unsweetened applesauce, mashed fresh banana, fresh berries with "sour cream," blended canned fruit or thickened frozen fruit or juice. To thicken frozen fruit or juice, heat, add cornstarch, arrowroot powder or flour blended with cold juice and stir over heat until thick. If necessary, blend dates with the thickening solution or use unsweetened frozen apple, pear or pineapple concentrate to add sweetening. If you want to "gild the lily" and serve a dessert-like waffle, top the "topping" with a scoop of frozen banana smoothie.

Apple-Oat Muffins

1 c. unpeeled raw apple, shredded (packed)
1 ½ c. rolled oats

1 c. raisins or chopped dates
½ t. salt
½ c. nuts, chopped

Combine and let stand to absorb moisture. Mix with fingers or fork and spoon into teflon muffin pans. Bake at 350 degrees for about 25 minutes or until lightly browned.

Granola

13 c. rolled oats
2 c. unsweetened coconut
1 c. fine nut meal
1 t. salt

1 c. wheat germ or cornmeal
2 c. whole wheat flour
1 c. chopped almonds
3 T. vanilla

1 c. or more as needed of water or fruit juice to moisten

Combine dry ingredients. Add water or fruit juice and vanilla and mix with fingers until moisture is evenly distributed but not too wet. Spread on cookie sheets or deeper baking pans about ½ inch thick and bake in preheated oven for 30 minutes at 300 degrees. Stir and decrease heat to 250 degrees until the cereal is crisp but only *slightly* brown. Stir and trade positions of pans as needed to brown evenly. When almost crisp, oven may be turned off and pans left to complete drying. You may want to refrigerate this cereal unless it is to be used within a few weeks, because the nuts could become rancid, especially in warm weather.

Variation: Blending the coconut and nut meal with the water or juice may spread the natural oil through the ingredients better to make them more tender, but we like the crunchiness of a harder cereal. Also some cooks like to blend 1 ½ c. of dates in the water or juice for sweetening, but instead we like to add date nuggets, raisins, sliced bananas, berries or other fresh, canned, frozen or stewed dried fruit to the cereal when we eat it. After adding juice, milk or yogurt for liquid, it resembles the museli used so widely in Europe.

Rice-Nut Milk

1 c. well-cooked brown rice
3 or 4 softened, pitted dates
¼ t. salt

½ c. cashews (sterilized)
2 c. water
1 t. vanilla

Blend all ingredients until smooth. Dilute with more water as desired. Stir well just before using.

Variations: Cooked oatmeal may be substituted for the rice and blanched almonds for the cashews. Instead of dates and water, you may experiment with unsweetened apple, pear or pineapple juice. Do not expect these "milks" to taste like dairy milk. They are simply a nutritious way to eat cereals as we have become accustomed, but with an alteration in the taste buds. It is not as hard as you may think.

Sweets

Smoothies

1 c. water, unsweetened fruit juice or nut milk
Ripe, peeled, frozen bananas, cut in chunks *or*
Fresh bananas and ice, using less liquid

Put liquid in blender and add chunks of banana while blades are whirling until the mixture is thick but not too heavy for the blender. A short time in the freezer before using will make the mixture more like ice cream, but because of its low fat content (not like commercial), it becomes very hard when left too long. For a sundae, top with fruit sauce and nuts. For carob ice cream, add carob powder and blend.

Variations: For a more sherbet-like texture, fruit juice is better while nut milk or even nonfat dry milk will make it more like ice cream. Combining one or more kinds of frozen berries or fruit with the bananas and different juices makes various delightful flavors.

We usually buy bananas on sale. Sometimes stores sell them cheaply when they are ripe in order to keep them from becoming overripe and spoiling. We peel them and put them in tight plastic bags. If the freezer is set at zero they will retain their light color, but should not be kept more than a few weeks.

Banana-Nut Cookies

1 c. rice-nut milk	6 mashed bananas
3 c. rolled oats	1 ½ c. w.w. flour
2 c. chopped nuts	2 t. vanilla
2 c. chopped dates or raisins	1 t. salt

Mix oats and flour. Add remaining ingredients and mix well. Drop by spoonful on teflon cookie sheet and bake at 325 degrees until lightly browned. Chewy and moist.

Fruit Candy

½ c. walnut meal	½ c. pecan meal
½ c. unsweetened coconut	1 c. dates, blended to a paste

1 t. vanilla, orange flavoring, mint flavoring or carob powder to taste may be added to all or to portions, if desired

Blend coconut until fine but not meal. Mix all ingredients well and add just enough water to form small balls.

Variations: Some may be rolled in finely chopped walnuts and/or coconut. Or some may be formed into a log, rolled in walnuts and/or coconut, chilled in refrigerator and then sliced. Must be refrigerated to keep and may be frozen.

SEASONINGS

Cinnamon Substitute

1–3 parts coriander seed and 1 part sweet anise seed or
1–3 parts coriander seed and 1 part cardamon

Grind together in moulinex or pulverize with mortar and pestle. Store in airtight container.

Chili Powder Substitute

2 T. paprika
1 T. dried green pepper
½ t. sweet basil
¼ t. ea. dill weed/savory/garlic
  powder

1 T. ea. parsley flakes/cumin
1 t. ea. oregano/onion powder
2 bay leaves

Grind in moulinex or blender.

Non-Irritating Curry Powder

1 T. ea. ground coriander/cumin/turmeric/
1 t. ea. garlic powder/salt
Mix and store in air-tight container.

Chicken-Like Seasoning

½ c. flaked food yeast
2 T. ea. onion powder/celery salt/parsley flakes/turmeric/salt
½ t. ea. sweet paprika/sage/rosemary/marjoram/savory

Mix thoroughly. Store in air-tight container and use as you would commercial chicken-style seasoning.

Salt Substitute

2 t. garlic powder
1 t. anise seed, finely ground
1 t. powdered lemon rind or dry lemon juice

1 t. basil
1 t. oregano

Store in a glass container. Add rice to prevent caking. Recipe from the U.S. Food and Drug Administration.

ADDENDUM:

MAKING SENSE OUT OF CALCIUM AND OSTEOPOROSIS

One of our dearest friends who was the picture of health fell not long ago and broke her hip. And the force of the fall on her shoulder also broke her collarbone. She could not explain the fall; she did not recall slipping or stumbling. Her doctor gave her the answer: "You did not break your hip because you fell; you fell because you broke your hip!"

"What?" she asked.

"Your hip bones just gave out. We call it 'Osteoporosis.'"

This may not be a new story to you, but we want it to be a story that does not have to be repeated unnecessarily for generations to come, and just at a time in life when our physical balance becomes less sure. Yet this condition has its beginnings early in life. Like any health scare, osteoporosis has brought us "therapies," ranging from genuine specialists to quacks and charlatans. Many millions of dollars are being spent on touting calcium additive pills, most of them doubtful at best.

So, because of the urgency and pervasiveness of this problem we have asked some of America's finest public health physicans and students of nutrition, to give us an authoritative statement on this crippling "disease." We have written it in a way to inform both laymen and physicians. No analysis will please all people, but this is one of the best we have seen on osteoporosis. Don't hesitate to use your dictionary or show this chapter to any careful medical doctor. Ask him what *he* thinks.

If you think taking calcium pills is all you need, you are one of those who need this most. Professor Robert P. Heaney specializes in mineral research and calcium absorption at Nebraska's Creighton University. Recently he warned that an increasing number of other nutrients may be hampered when calcium is taken in excess: "With supplements you are getting a high dose of calcium, rather than the natural balance of many nutrients found in food. This dosage may in turn upset the balance of other nutrients in the body such as iron and zinc."

Size of the Problem

Osteoporosis affects 15–20 million persons in the United States.[1] Osteoporosis is more common in older women than strokes, heart attacks, diabetes, breast cancer or rheumatoid arthritis. It affects 25% of women after a natural menopause and 50% after removal of ovaries without estrogen replacement.[2] The annual cost of this disease is $3.8 billion.[1]

About 1.3 million fractures due to this occur each year in people 45 years of age or older. It is estimated that 90% of all fractures past age 60 are due to osteoporosis.[3] Also 5.3% of all hospitalized patients over age 65 have fracture as their diagnosis and 10.2% over age 85. After age 85, 4% of the population suffers a fracture each year.[3]

There are 200,000 hip fractures a year. A white woman has a 15% lifetime risk of a hip fracture. Half of the hip fractures occur after the age of 80.[4] After one hip fracture the risk of it happening in the other hip is twenty times more likely.[2] Female to male ratio for femur neck fractures is five to one but only two to one for the trochanteric (hip) fractures.[5] Mortality within the first year of a hip fracture runs about 20% making these fractures the twelfth leading cause of death.

Vertebral fractures occur in about 5% of white women by age 70.[4] By age 80 most white women will have x-ray signs of at least one vertebral partial compression. Some say that 50% of white women by age 65 have detectable vertebral wedging which occurs before the vertebra totally collapses.[2] Under 75 years of age the Colles fracture (distal forearm) is the commonest fracture to occur.[4] After age 50 wrist fractures are ten times more frequent in women than men.[2]

Osteoporosis is a major problem of older women.[6] But women should not wait until the menopause to take estrogens to prevent the problem. They must do something in the early years of life to prevent the disease. First there needs to be a good diet and second a good exercise program to develop peak bone mass during childhood. Then in the 30's exercise should still be continued. Some would also suggest insuring adequate calcium intake. According to some the glass of milk a day does not give enough added calcium in the United States but even without any milk peoples of many parts of the world do well. Walking, jogging, bicycling, or any aerobic exercise should be a part of the lifestyle.

What Is Osteoporosis?

"Primary osteoporosis is an age-related disorder characterized by decreased bone mass and by increased susceptibility to fractures in the absence of other recognizable causes of bone loss."[1]

Two types of bone exist. Compact cortical bone forms the outer lining of skeletal bones. Trabecular or medullary bone forms plates that traverse the internal cavities of the skeleton. The proportion of one type to the other varies depending upon the site. Vertebral bones are primarily of the trabecular type while the long bones like the femur are mostly the cortical type. The responses of the two types to metabolic influences and their risk of having a fracture differ.

Bone is constantly being resorbed and formed again throughout life. Various factors, such as hormones, mechanical and electrical forces, etc. influence this constant reforming of the bones. Osteoclasts are bone-resorbing cells. Osteoblasts are bone-forming cells. They produce the collagen matrix of the bone. About ten days after the collagen matrix is put in place the calcium and phosphorus crystals are laid down, a process called mineralization. The cycle of resorbing the bone and building new bone takes 3–4 months. Adults have 10–30% of the bone replaced each year in this remodeling process.[2]

Peak bone mass is achieved at about 35 years of age for cortical bone and earlier for trabecular bone. Sex, race, nutrition, exercise, and overall health influence peak mass. After reaching its peak, bone mass declines throughout life because of an imbalance in remodeling. Bones lose both mineral and organic matrix. This loss is enhanced in a number of diseases. Bone loss occurs at the rate of 0.5% per year from age 35–40 and on but increases to 1% after the menopause for the next ten years.[27] This means a negative calcium balance will exist of 25 mg a day and after the menopause of 50 mg a day.[3]

Up until about 50 both men and women lose bone mass slowly. However, women lose bone rapidly in the first 5–6 years following menopause. Their loss at this time is about six times that of men. They lose about as much bone during this period as they got during adolescence following the hormonal surges.[2] At 65 years of age women and men lose bone at an equal rate. But by age 80 a woman will have lost 47% of her trabecular bone and a man only 14%.[2]

Many diseases increase the risk of osteoporosis. The reasons for this are not known. Diabetics are more prone to get osteoporosis, and particularly at the ankle, an uncommon site for the nondiabetic osteoporotic.[5] Rheumatoid arthritics and those with chronic lung disease are at higher risk of osteoporosis. Lactose intolerance may also increase the risk probably because of low calcium intake and absorption. Use of steroids may increase the risk for the arthritic. Chronic lung disease patients—among others—may have a higher risk because of their cigarette smoking.

Those Who Are Susceptible

The clinical picture helps to establish the diagnosis of osteoporosis.

Although osteoporosis may occur in any bone, fractures do occur more commonly in specific areas. They occur in the vertebrae between T-8 and L-3. These occur more commonly in women than in men. Loss of height or development of kyphosis may occur. It is said that transparent skin (check the back of the hands) is more common in people with osteoporosis.[2] Opaque skin is 35% thicker than transparent skin.

People with rheumatoid arthritis tend to have a greater risk of osteoporosis. This may be partially due to use of cortisone which increases risk.[2]

Loss of teeth may be due to osteoporosis of the jaw bones and may be an indication of higher risk of problems with other bones. However, loss of teeth is more commonly due to other causes.

Blood and urine tests are of no value in making the diagnosis of osteoporosis but may be useful in ruling out secondary causes.

Cause

Osteoporosis correlates with the decline in bone mass with age. Women are at twice the risk as men as bone mass is 30% higher in men. Whites are at greater risk than blacks. Blacks have 10% greater bone mass. However, contrary to the consensus thinking a recent report states that hip fracture rates were no different in black and white men and even black women.[7] It did show white women had twice the risk of black women. The reason for this is that their incidence rates began to rise five years earlier than with black women.

Women with ancestors from Africa or the Mediterranean area or Hispanics are not as prone to osteoporosis as those descendants of people from northern Europe, China, or Japan.[2] Swedes appear to be larger boned than Italians and yet do have a higher incidence of osteoporosis.

Rapid bone turnover or reduced bone formation have been documented in osteoporosis patients. Some studies suggest it begins *before* menopause.[8] Some insist it starts *after*.[9] In either event, it is mostly a woman's disease.[8, 10]

Prevention

Prevention has been revolving around the perimenopausal period but probably should be around developing adequate peak skeletal mass by proper habits during adolescence and childhood. Studies show that milk drinking in childhood may result in higher bone density decades later in menopause.[11] Slimming of adolescent girls on needless diets before the peak bone mass has been achieved may be detrimental.[12] Small people with little bone mass to start with are at greater risk of osteoporosis.

A. Exercise. Exercise is important. It is the only known measure which will not only reduce bone breakdown but increase bone formation. It is said to produce electrical potentials in the bone which stimulates new bone growth.[2] Women who exercise are said to have higher levels of estrogens and lower levels of adrenal hormones which favors bone formation.[2]

Inactivity leads to bone loss. Some recent studies suggest that weight-bearing exercise may reduce bone loss. Modest weight-bearing exercise, such as walking, is recommended. Bone density is greater in the right hand of right-handed people but greater in the left hand of left-handed people. The frequency of the exercise is more important to bone stimulus than the peak strain achieved.

Swimming or ordinary calisthenics are good for joint mobility but have little effect on bone mass.[13] It has been suggested swimming may be useful for those who already have osteoporosis since it will not put much of a strain on an already weakened skeletal system.[2]

Taking calcium supplements without increasing exercise is like neglecting half the treatment. Calcium acts to suppress bone resorption whereas mechanical stress seems to enhance bone formation. Combining the two measures seems to be the most practical approach.[13]

One study showed postmenopausal women (mean age 53) who exercised one hour three times a week increased their total body calcium (a measure of bone mass) by 2.6% over a one-year period, while in the control group of sedentary women total-body calcium decreased by 2.4%.[13] Some suggest the principal underlying reason for bone loss with age is considered to be a decline in physical activity. Exercise may also be beneficial by preserving one's muscular coordination and reducing the risk of falls.

Physicians treating patients in general as well as those who treat patients with fractures do recognize the benefits of rapid return to function and the avoidance of prolonged immobilization. Immobilization and bed rest produce rapid bone loss (1% per week), while exercise involving weight bearing reduces bone loss and increases bone mass. It is interesting that parathyroidectomy prevents immobilization bone loss.[14]

Studies of patients on partial bed rest at the Public Health Service Hospital in San Francisco did show that quiet standing for three hours a day had a somewhat positive effect on calcium metabolic balance and on the measured density of the os calcis. Ambulation for four hours a day prevented calcium loss even if the remaining 20 hours a day were spent in bed.[13]

Exercise which induces amenorrhea in young women may lead to increased bone loss. This may be because they have so little fat, they are producing very little estrogen.

During yearly seasons of unusual activity there are also more fractures occurring. For example, in England it is reported hospitals get more fractures during December and January during the busy shopping season.[15] In Jerusalem women have more fractures at the time of preparation for the Jewish festivals.[15] Yet, the March and April rise in occurrence may be due to the vitamin D levels being lowest at this time of the year.[15]

B. Estrogens. [17,22,23,24,25,26] For several years after the menopause, whether natural or induced, there is an acceleration of bone loss. Early menopause is one of the strongest predictors of osteoporosis. The common questionable practice of surgical removal of the ovaries when a hysterectomy is done greatly increases the risk of osteoporosis if estrogen replacement therapy is not done.

Young women with low levels of estrogen, or who are amenorrheic, or those who have had their ovaries removed have lower bone densities and a higher rate of fractures.[16,21]

Women who are underweight are at higher risk than those who are overweight. This may be due to the fact that fat tissue produces estrogens which are protective. These estrogens are produced from the androgens that come from the adrenal gland.[2] The greater weight or stress of the obese on the bones helps to develop better bones also. However, obese women have an excess risk of many cancers, so obesity is not something to be desired.

The contraceptive use of the "pill" may be protective also as the pill contains both estrogens and progestogen. Both of these hormones help the bones, possibly by stimulating the release of calcitonin which inhibits bone breakdown.[2]

Because of the high levels of estrogens in pregnancy, having children may be protective against osteoporosis. Progesterones also are high during pregnancy and this also is protective. One study in the United States found two-thirds of the women who had osteoporosis to be those who had no children.[2] However, in undernourished areas of the world the calcium supplies may be limited and pregnancy would have a deleterious effect on the bones.

Estrogens operate primarily through other hormones to control bone formation and breakdown by improving calcium balance. It blocks actions of parathyroid hormone. When there is little estrogen (menopause) the parathyroid hormone, even at low levels, affects the bones adversely.[2] High levels of estrogens (during pregnancy) stimulate the activation of vitamin D. Osteoporotic women are less able to activate vitamin D in the kidneys. Calcitonin, the bone-protecting hormone, is stimulated by estrogens.[2]

Studies have shown a substantial reduction in hip and wrist fractures in women whose estrogen replacement was begun within five years of menopause.[18] Studies suggest that estrogen lowers the risk of vertebral fractures. Even when begun six years after menopause, estrogen has been shown to prevent further bone loss. However, it will not restore it to premenopausal levels. Estrogen pills appear to be protective even at low doses, such as 0.625 mg of conjugated equine estrogen (25 ug of mestranol and 2 mg of estradiol valerate daily exemplify other protective regimens[1]). The longer the time of using estrogens the lower the fracture risk.[19] All studies have been based exclusively on white women.

A study was reported in 1976 of a group of women within three years of their menopause who had their ovaries removed.[2] To be most effective, it has been determined, estrogens must be given within three years of the menopause.[2,3] Those women who took estrogens had no bone loss compared to those on the placebo. Women who had estrogens for four years and then none the next four years lost as much bone as those who had not taken the estrogens. Estrogens must be taken until the natural slowing down of bone loss occurs, which is around the age of 65. Those who took it for eight years showed no bone loss.

Estrogen users have 60% less wrist and hip fractures and 90% less vertebral fractures.[2,6] Those who take estrogens even within five years of the menopause are four times more likely to remain free of wrist and hip fractures.[2]

Women who have had a natural menopause also should be considered for cyclic estrogen replacement if they have no contraindications and if they understand the risks and agree to regular medical examinations. The duration of estrogen therapy need not be limited.

There is no convincing evidence that initiating estrogen therapy in elderly women (over age 65) will prevent osteoporosis.[20]

Estrogen users have a greater risk of cancer of the lining of the uterus. Estrogen-associated endometrial cancer iş usually manifested at an early stage and is rarely fatal when managed properly. However, those using a progestogen in the cycle actually have a lower risk than women not on treatment.[2] Progestogen is protective. Women who don't ovulate and therefore don't produce progesterone, or obese women who produce more estrogens would be more prone to develop endometrial cancer. The increased risk of endometrial cancer with just use of estrogens is four to eight times that of women who don't take estrogens. For this reason, progestogen is important. There are over ten times as many dying from hip fractures as from endometrial cancer.

The bulk of the evidence indicates that estrogen use is not associated with an increased risk of breast cancer. Adding a progestogen probably reduces the risk of endometrial cancer, but there is little information about the safety of long-term combined estrogen and progestogen treatment in postmenopausal women.

Estrogens may increase the risk of hypertension. It may also increase the risk of blood clots. However, for older women after menopause estrogens actually decrease the risk of cardiovascular disease.[2]

Younger women on progestogens in oral contraceptives have a higher risk of hypertension and cardiovascular disease. Some progestogens may blunt or eliminate the favorable effects of estrogen on lipoproteins.

Some have suggested that since only 25% of women get osteoporosis and there is a risk to use of estrogens only those at high risk should take estrogens.[2] If bone mass could be measured twice a year one could tell who needs estrogens by this method. However, such diagnostic techniques are not yet available to everyone. High risk individuals are those whose ovaries have been removed, short women, thin women, or those with a strong family history of the disease. However, those who have had cancer of the female organs or a family history of it should not take estrogens.[2]

Until more data on risks and benefits are available physicians and patients may prefer to reserve estrogen (with or without progestogen) therapy for conditions that confer a high risk of osteoporosis, such as the occurrence of premature menopause.

For those who take estrogens, it is a long-term procedure with close followup by the physician, with examination of the breast and pelvic area yearly, at least, self-breast examination every month, and routine checking of your blood pressure. Some suggest an endometrial biopsy at the outset if you have not had a hysterectomy. The progesterone may cause menstrual-like bleeding. To avoid this some are recommending small doses of progesterone daily with the estrogen.[2]

C. Calcium and its sources.[30,31,33,34] Some believe it is likely that an increase in calcium intake to from 1000 to 1500 mg per day beginning well before the menopause will reduce the incidence of osteoporosis in postmenopausal women. They also believe it may prevent age related bone loss in men as well.

Elderly women absorb less calcium and also excrete it more readily through the kidneys.[13] Absorption is less in osteoporotics also.[27,28]

The major source of calcium in our diet is from milk. There are 291 mg per cup of skim milk, which is the preferred form of milk to minimize fat intake. For those unable to get their needs by diet, supplementation is recommended by some. In many places in the world average intake is less than 400 mg a day with no adverse effects. Total vegetarians get under 300 mg a day. A good food source other than dairy products is tofu (if precipitated out with calcium sulfate). A half pound will provide as much calcium as in a cup of milk. A cup of greens from turnips, mustard, or collards provides considerable amounts. Five oranges will give almost as much as in a cup of milk but it would take ten cups of orange juice to do the same. Nuts, grains and beans will supply some but not in large amounts. One can add powdered skim milk to all kinds of recipes to get more calcium into the diet.

Tums, the overcounter antacid tablets, are an inexpensive source of calcium.[6] Each tablet provides 200 mg calcium.

1200 mg tablets of calcium gluconate, lactate and carbonate contain 108, 156, and 480 mg of calcium respectively. Calcium carbonate has the lowest absorption rate of the three but is the least expensive.[20] Others state there is no evidence of any difference in absorption of the three.[29] Calcium carbonate requires less pills to meet one's needs but is more constipating. Lederle's Caltrate provides 600 mg calcium per tablet. OsCal 500 provides 500 mg calcium per tablet.

Calcium supplementation should not go above the recommended levels of between 1000 and 1500 mg a day because of the risk of urinary tract stones according to the 1984 NIH Consensus Development Conference on Osteoporosis.[1] Anyone with a history of kidney stones should undertake calcium supplementation only with the guidance of a physician. Excess intake of calcium will result in excess kidney excretion and therefore greater risk of kidney stones. Some suggest using thiazides to keep the calcium from being excreted and reducing the risk of kidney stones.[32]

What is not known is the rate of complications resulting from raising women's calcium intake. Until we have better information it may be wise to recommend increased calcium intake only for those at high risk (premature menopause, thin, family history of osteoporosis, smoking, and alcohol use) and who do not have obvious contraindications such as hyperparathyroidism or hypercalciuria.[32]

Calcium, once absorbed, suppresses parathyroid hormone secretion. It is this hormone which controls bone remodeling.[2] The absorption of calcium may be more important than how much calcium one gets.[35]

Fiber, however, is a factor.[36] Cereal fiber tends to decrease absorption more than fruit or vegetable fiber. For this reason those taking calcium tablets may better take them one hour before meals or two hours after meals. Some have even suggested not using high fiber foods in the meals that contain large amounts of calcium.[2]

Stress may decrease the absorption of calcium by 30%. It also increases the production of adrenal hormones which stimulate bone breakdown. So stress has an adverse effect upon the bones.

Fat can decrease the absorption of calcium but only in the presence of steatorrhea.[36] Lactose does increase the absorption. During states of increased need such as calcium deficiency, pregnancy, lactation, there is an increased absorption. There is decreased absorption with vitamin D deficiency, during menopause and in old age. In many disease states there is a decrease in calcium absorption. Stressful situations may reduce absorption and also increase urinary excretion of calcium.[35] Ensure (60% glucose polymer and 40% sucrose) increased calcium absorption in test meals from 1.5 to 5 times what was ordinarily absorbed in patients. Those with the poorest absorption had the greatest increase with Ensure.[37]

D. Calcium to Phosphorus Ratio.[41] A poor *calcium to phosphorus ratio* has been shown to reduce the intestinal absorption of calcium in small animals.[38] Therefore either a low calcium intake or a high phosphorus intake may cause the same problem. The ideal ratio as recommended by the Food and Nutrition Board of the National Research Council is 1:1 except for in the first year of life where infants are started at a 1.5:1 ideal ratio. However, hardly anyone in the United States gets a 1:1 ratio except for infants because that is about the ratio in milk. Ratios in American diets are from 1:2.8 up to 1:4. Osteoporosis has been produced in monkeys with a ratio of 1:5.[39]

Phosphorus is being added to many foods in the processing. It will be found in processed meats, cheeses, soft drinks, and food starches. This may increase the intake by 0.5 to 1.0 gram a day.[38] With an elimination of these foods (soft drinks, meat) one may get his ratio to the recommended level.

E. *Vitamin D.*[43,44,45,46] Vitamin D is required for optimal calcium absorption. The requirements increase with age. Persons who do not get adequate daily sunlight, such as those confined to home or to a nursing facility, are at special risk for vitamin D deficiency. Vitamin D has dangerous effects at high doses. The toxic dose varies with individuals but has occurred as low as 2000–5000 IU daily. No one should consume more than 15 to 20 ug (600 to 800 IU, twice the daily RDA) without a doctor's recommendation.

Vitamin D is made in the skin and eaten in our foods. Then it is converted in the liver to 25 hydroxy-vitamin D (25 OHD). This in the kidney is transformed to 1,25 dihydroxy-vitamin D often noted as 1,25 $(OH)_2D$. This is the active form which is needed to assist in calcium absorption as well as for metabolism of the bone.

F. *Fluoride.*[47] Fluoride in association with calcium may have a role in treatment of severe cases but its safety and efficacy are unproved. Prospective studies are under way to determine this point.

G. *High Protein Intake.* In a study of 320 lacto-ovo-vegetarians who had been on this diet for 20 years versus 320 omnivorous males 20–79 years of age there was no difference in bone density.[48] However, studies of women showed much poorer density in omnivores than in vegetarians.[49] This may be due to the higher protein intake with more sulfur amino acids which causes a reduction in renal tubular reabsorption of calcium.[50] Although urinary calcium excretion is increased with a higher intake of protein, intestinal absorption is also increased.

Vegetarian women between the ages of 50 and 89 lose only 18% of their bone mass whereas nonvegetarians lose 35% even with the same amount of calcium in their diets.[2]

It has been suggested that a high acid ash diet stimulates osteoclastic bone resorption and increases urinary calcium.[51] Meat is a high acid ash food. In rats long-term ingestion of excess acid causes osteoporosis. To protect the body from acidosis the bone is resorbed to provide more calcium and phosphate to maintain blood pH.

Meat has a low calcium to phosphorus ratio which could be another reason for the problem among nonvegetarians.

Although there is considerable scientific argument over whether or not dietary protein increases urinary calcium excretion, there is no argument over the fact that vegetarian women have less osteoporosis. The reasons for this are being sought.

H. *Alcohol.*[40] Bones of young chronic alcoholics were similar in weight to postmenopausal patients. Fractures and osteoporosis have been noted in alcoholics. A study of women aged 20–35 showed bone mass negatively and significantly associated with alcohol consumption.[52] Alcohol often displaces good foods in the diet. High amounts hinder calcium absorption and may be toxic to the bone cells. Even social drinkers have 2½ times the risk of osteoporosis as nondrinkers.[53] No studies have been done to see what one or two drinks a day might do. Possible mechanisms as to how alcohol increases osteoporosis risk have been suggested.[40]

I. *Vitamin A.* Excess vitamin A or D accelerate bone resorption and should be avoided.[20] Vitamin A is said to stimulate bone loss.[2] However, it is doubtful this would apply to carotene. The body does not convert carotene to vitamin A if it has sufficient vitamin A. Carotene comes only from plant sources and is nontoxic. Animal products or vitamin pills containing large amounts of vitamin A should be avoided.

J. Aluminum Antacids. Aluminum antacids may be a factor in increasing osteoporosis risk.[40] These increase calcium excretion. Such are Amphojel, Di-gel, Gelusil, Maalox, Mylanta, and Rolaids. Alka-Seltzer, Tums, and Citrocarbonate do not contain aluminum.

K. Other Drugs. The cortisone type of drugs cause severe bone loss, often of the ribs.[2] Anticonvulsants increase production of enzymes which inactivate vitamin D leading to less calcium absorption.[2] Thyroid above three grains a day seems to produce bone loss just like hyperthyroidism does.[2] Diuretics, as furosemide increase calcium excretion but thiazides reduce the calcium lost in the urine.[2]

L. Sodium. Sodium increases the excretion of calcium.[2] With the increased excretion of calcium blood calcium is lowered. The parathyroid hormone then causes the calcium to come from the bones to bring the blood calcium back up to normal. This produces osteoporosis.

There was no change in urinary calcium with 200 mg of sodium but an increase in excretion at 2000 mg. One teaspoonful of salt gives one that much. There are no studies as to what happens at higher levels. At least it would be wise to keep down to the U.S. Dietary Goals of no more than one added teaspoonful of salt a day. That means we need to lower the intake of salt to about one-third what most of us get.

M. Coffee. Coffee decreases the absorption of iron and calcium. With iron it is appreciable. With calcium it is a very small amount but over a lifetime is considered a risk factor for osteoporosis. One study showed 31% of osteoporotic women drank four or more cups of coffee a day while only 19% of those not having this condition drank that much.[2]

N. Preventive Strategies. Strategies to prevent falls must be developed particularly for those who may fall because of use of specific drugs. Sleeping pills or barbitruates may cause dizziness. Environmental interventions can minimize home hazards that increase the chances of falling. Correctable impairment of visual acuity may be an important preventive step. For the elderly, those over 80, who may already have osteoporosis, measures to prevent falls may be more important than the treatment of the osteoporosis.

O. Cigarette Smoking.[54,23] Cigarette smoking increases the risk in both men and women. Women who smoke reach menopause several years earlier than nonsmokers. Smokers may be less obese and therefore have lower estrogen levels. They may have a lower peak bone mass because of smoking early in life. Smokers have an earlier menopause. All these could be factors increasing the smoker's risk of osteoporosis.

Recommendations[56,57,58,59,60]

Treatment is primarily one of prevention. The proven prophylaxis is exercise which must be against gravity such as jogging, not swimming. High risk individuals cannot be selected by x-ray appearance because bone loss cannot be noted until at least 30% is lost. High risk persons such as those with malabsorptive states, lactase deficiency, or inflammatory bowel disease could receive oral calcium supplements.[55]

If one discovers osteoporosis has already developed, an exercise program should be started (with caution), stop smoking, stop drinking alcohol and coffee, and lower the intake of salt. Of course, these things should have been done earlier to prevent the disease.

1. The best form of treatment is prevention.

2. Prevention means developing peak bone mass in childhood and adolescence. This means good nutrition and a weight-bearing exercise program.

3. A weight-bearing exercise program throughout life is important.

4. Avoid deleterious substances such as tobacco, alcohol, tea, or coffee.

5. Stay on a vegetarian diet. Avoid meat.

6. Avoid soft drinks.

7. Avoid commonly used unnecessary medications.

8. Get adequate sunshine.

9. Develop a lifestyle which allows you to cope adequately with stress.

10. A very high risk individual (thin, small, family history) may choose to use estrogens in combination with progesterone at menopause.

11. Keep on a low salt diet.

12. Additional calcium is probably not needed if one decreases intake of phosphorus and sodium and is on a vegetarian diet and gets adequate exercise.

The percent of our calcium and phosphorus intakes from various food groups is as follows:[42]

Food Group	Calcium	Phosphorus
Meat, poultry, fish	4.2	28.0
Eggs	2.3	4.3
Dairy products (excluding butter)	74.5	34.2
Citrus Fruits	1.2	0.9
Non-citrus fruits	1.4	1.3
Potatoes & sweet potatoes	1.1	3.7
Dark-green, deep yellow vegetables	1.4	0.7
Other vegetables including tomatoes	4.8	4.8
Dry beans, peas, nuts, soy products	3.0	6.3
Grain products	3.7	13.1

Bibliography

1. Robert P. Heaney, M.D., in a speech before a symposium sponsored by the California Dietetic Association. Reported by Rose Dosti in *The Los Angeles Times*, March 20, 1986.

2. Notelovitz M, Ware M: *Stand Tall! Every Woman's Guide to Preventing Osteoporosis*. Bantam Books, New York, 1982.

3. Recker RR: Osteoporosis. Contemporary Nutrition 8 (No. 5): May, 1983.

4. Cummings SR, Nevitt MC, Haber RJ: Prevention of osteoporosis and osteoporotic fractures. Western Journal of Medicine 13: 684–687, 1985.

5. Ahronheim JC: Osteoporosis in the elderly. Practical Gastroenterology 8 (No. 5): 41–52, 1984.

6. Cancila C: Age-related diseases preventable now. *American Medical News*, 9–10, June 1, 1984.

7. Doepel LK: Looking at menopause's role in osteoporosis. JAMA 254: 2379–2380, 1985.

8. Riggs BL, Wahner HW, Dunn WL, Mazess RB, Offord KP: Differential changes in bone mineral density of the appendicular and axial skeleton with aging. J Clin Invest 67:328–335.

9. Richelson LS, Wahner HW, Melton L III, Riggs BL: Relative contributions of aging and estrogen deficiency to postmenopausal bone loss. N Engl J Med 311: 1273–1275, 1984.

10. Dequeker J, Geusens P: Contributions of aging and estrogen deficiency to postmenopausal bone loss. N Engl J Med 313: 453, 1985.

11. Sandler RB, Slemenda CW, LaPorte RE, Cauley JA, Schramm MM, Barresi ML, Kriska AM: Postmenopausal bone density and milk consumption in childhood and adolescence. Am J Clin Nutr 42: 270–274, 1985.

12. Hausman P: *The Calcium Bible*. Rawson Associates, New York, 1984.

13. Korcok M: Add exercise to calcium for osteoporosis prevention. JAMA 247:1106–1107, 1982.

14. Draper HH, Bell RR: Nutrition and osteoporosis. In: Draper HH (editor): *Advances in Nutritional Research*, vol. 2, Plenum Publishing Corporation, 1979.

15. Evans JG: Undernutrition and femoral fracture. Lancet 1: 710, 1983.

16. Klibanski A, Neer RM, Beitins IZ, Ridgway EC, Zervas NT, McArthur JW: Decreased bone density in hyperproteinemic women. N Engl J Med 303: 1511–1514, 1980.

17. Horsman A, Jones M, Francis R, Nordin C: The effect of estrogen dose on postmenopausal bone loss. N Engl J Med 309: 1405–1407, 1983.

18. Nutrition Reviews: Estrogens given after the menopause protect against fractures. Nutr Rev 38: 80, 1980.

19. Johnson RE, Specht EE: The risk of hip fracture in postmenopausal females with and without estrogen drug exposure. Am J Pub Health 71: 138–144, 1981.

20. Nutrition & the M.D.: Calcium supplementation in adult women. Nutrition & the M.D. 11 (No. 3): 1–3, 1985.

21. Hale WE, Stewart RB, Marks RG: Thiazide and fractures of bones. Ltr to the editor. N Engl J Med 310: 926–927, 1984.

22. Silberner J: Estrogen use raises questions. *Science News* 128: 279–280, 1985.

23. Wilson PWF, Garrison RJ, Castelli WP: Postmenopausal estrogen use, cigarette

smoking, and cardiovascular morbidity in women over 50. N Engl J Med 313: 103801040, 1985.

24. Stampfer MJ, Willett WC, Colditz GA, Rosner B, Speizer FE, Hennekens CH: A prospective study of postmenopausal estrogen therapy and coronary heart disease. N Engl J Med 313: 1044–1049, 1985.

25. Bailar JC III: When research results are in conflict. N Engl J Med 313: 1080–1081, 1985.

26. Shapiro S, Kelly JP, Rosenberg L, Kaufman DW, Helmrich SP, Rosenshein NB, Lewis JL, Knapp RC, Stolley PD, Schottenfeld D: Risk of localized and widespread endometrial cancer in relation to recent and discontinued use of conjugated estrogens. N Engl J Med 969–972, 1985.

27. Whedon DG: Osteoporosis. N Engl J Med 305: 397–399, 1981.

28. Yano K, Heilbrun LK, Wasnich RD, Hankin JH, Vogel JM: The relationship between diet and bone mineral content of multiple skeletal sites in elderly Japanese-American men and women living in Hawaii. Am J Clin Nutr 42: 877–888, 1985.

29. Nutrition Action: Calcium redux. *Nutrition Action*, 12–13, December, 1984.

30. Walker ARP, Walker BF: Recommended dietary allowances and third world populations. Am J Clin Nutr 34: 2319–2321, 1981.

31. Heaney RP, Gallagher JC, Johnston CC, Neer R, Parfitt AM, BChir MB, Whedon GD: Calcium nutrition and bone health in the elderly. Am J Clin Nutr 36: 986–1013, 1982.

32. Heath H III: Calcium supplementation and risk of renal calculi. JAMA 254: 964, 1985.

33. Wasnich RD, Benfante RJ, Yano K, Heilburn L, Vogel JM: Thiazide effect on the mineral content of bone. N Engl J Med 309: 344–347, 1983.

34. Nutrition Reviews: Calcium: How much is too much? Nutr Rev 43: 345–346, 1985.

35. Irwin MI, Kienholz EW: A conspectus of research on calcium requirements of man. In Irwin MI (editor): Nutritional Requirements of Man. The Nutrition Foundation, Washington, D.C. 1980, 135–212.

36. Allen LH: Calcium bioavailability and absorption: a review. Am J Clin Nutr 35:783–808, 1982.

37. Nutrition & the M.D.: Effect of meal composition on calcium absorption. Nutrition & the M.D. vol. 11 (No. 11), 1985.

38. Linkswiler HM, Zemel MB: Calcium to phosphorus ratios. Contemporary Nutrition 4 (No. 5): May 1979.

39. Lutwak L: Current concepts of bone metabolism. Ann Int Med 80: 630–644, 1974.

40. Spencer H, Kramer L, Osis D: Factors contributing to calcium loss in aging. Am J Clin Nutr 36: 776–787, 1982.

41. Meyers FH, Jawetz E, Goldfein A: Review of Medical Pharmacology p. 356, Lange Medical Publications, Los Altos, California, 1974.

42. U.S. Department of Agriculture: Contribution of major food groups to nutrient levels. National Food Review 29. 7, Winter–Spring Issue, 1985.

43. Nordin BEC, Baker MR, Horsman A, Peacock M: A prospective trial of the effect of vitamin D supplementation on metacarpal bone loss in elderly women. Am J Clin Nutr 42: 470–474, 1985.

44. Slovik DM, Adams JS, Neer RM, Holick MF, Potts JT: Deficient Production of 1,25-dihydroxyvitamin D in elderly osteoporotic patients. N Engl J Med 305: 372–374, 1981.

45. Omdahl JL, Gary PJ, Hunsaker LA, Hunt WC, Goodwin JS: Nutritional status in a healthy elderly population: vitamin D. Am J Clin Nutr 36: 1225–1233, 1982.

46. Parfitt AM, BChir MB, Gallagher JC, Heaney RP, Johnston CC, Neer R, Whedon D: Vitamin D and bone health in the elderly. Am J Clin Nutr 36: 1014–1031, 1982.

47. Madans J, Kleinman JC, Cornoni-Huntley J: The relationship between hip fracture and water fluoridation: An analysis of national data. Am J Pub Health 73: 296–298, 1983.

48. Marsh AG, Sanchez TV, Chaffee FL, Mayor GH, Mickelsen O: Bone mineral mass in adult lacto-ovo-vegetarian and omnivorous males. Am J Clin Nutr 37: 453–456, 1983.

49. Marsh AG, Sanchez TV, Mickelsen O, Keiser J, Mayor G: Cortical bone density of adult lacto-ovo-vegetarian and omnivorous women. J Am Diet Assoc 76: 148–151, 1980.

50. Nutrition Reviews: High protein diets and bone homeostasis. Nutr Rev 39: 11–13, 1981.

51. Barzel US: Osteoporosis in young men. Arch Int Med 142: 2079–2080, 1982.

52. Sowers MF, Wallace RB, Lemke JH: Correlates of forearm bone mass among women during maximal bone mineralization. Prev Med 14: 585–596, 1985.

53. Nutrition Action: Losers Weepers. *Nutrition Action* July/August 1985.

54. Jensen J, Christiansen C, Rodbro P: Cigarette smoking, serum estrogens, and bone loss during hormone-replacement therapy early after menopause. N Engl J Med 313: 973–975, 1985.

55. Kantrowitz FW: Therapy for post-menopausal osteoporosis. Int Med Alert pp. 19–20, March 15, 1982.

56. Nicholas JA, Wilson PD: Diagnosis and treatment of osteoporosis. JAMA 171: 2279–2284, 1959.

57. Heaney RP: Early postmenopausal osteoporosis. JAMA 249: 90, 1983.

58. Riggs BL, Seeman E, Hodgson SF, Taves DR, O'Fallon WM: Effect of the fluoride/calcium regimen in vertebral fracture occurrence in postmenopausal osteoporosis. N Engl J Med 306: 446–450, 1982.

59. Woodard D: Treatment of osteoporosis. Ltr. to the editor. N Engl J Med 312: 647, 1985.

60. Kanis JA: Treatment of osteoporotic fracture. Lancet 1: 27–32, 1984.

NOTES

Chapter 2
1. "Update," *New Wine*, January 1979, 24–29.
2. Ern Baxter, *I Almost Died*. Integrity House, P.O. Box Z. Mobile, AL 36616.
3. Philippians 3:20, NIV.
4. Romans 8:14–17.
5. Revelation 3:20–21; 1:6; 5:10.
6. 1 Corinthians 3:16–17.
7. 1 Corinthians 10:31.
8. 3 John 2.
9. Proverbs 17:22.
10. J. T. Fisher and Lowell S. Hawley, *A Few Buttons Missing*. J. B. Lippincott, Philadelphia, 1951.

Chapter 3
1. David G. Jose and Robert A. Good. Immune resistance and malnutrition. *Lancet* 1:314, 1972.
2. 1 Corinthians 10:31.
3. Reported in *USA Today*, April 5, 1985.
4. Harris, Robert S., H. V. Loesecke. *Nutritional Evaluation of Food Processing*. Westport, Connecticut, AVI Publishing Co., In., 1971, 419.
5. Sheets, O., O. A. Leonard, M. Geiger. *Food Res*. 6:553, 1941.

Chapter 4
1. Tufts University Diet and Nutrition Letter 1:1, March 1983.
2. J. A. Scharffenberg, "Natural versus refined sugar." *Adventist Review*, June 20, 1985. 7.

3. Journal of American Dental Association, Sept., 1955.
4. Steinman, R. R., J. Leonora and R. J. Singh. The Effect of Desalivation Upon Pulpal Function and Dental Caries in Rats. *Journal of Dental Research* 59:176–185, 1980.
5. Nizel, A. E. Carbohydrates—Dental Caries Promotion. *Nutrition in Preventive Dentistry*. 2nd edition, 53–80. W. B. Saunders. Philadelphia 1981.
6. Shaw, J. H., E. A. Sweeney, C. C. Cappuccino, et al. "Cariology." *Textbook of Oral Biology*. W. B. Saunders, Philadelphia, 1978. 955–973.
7. Ibid.
8. Sognnaes, R. F. "Caries-conducive Effect of a Purified Diet When Fed to Rodents During Tooth Development." Journal Southern California State Association., 28:367, 1960.
9. Crane, Milton G., M.D., HEALTH AND HEALING, Winter 1983/84, 16–20. Henry A. Schroeder, *Trace Elements in Man*, Devin-Adair Co., Old Greenwich, CN, 1973. University of Missouri Annual Conference on Trace Elements.
10. Weimar Institute Lectures (Newstart Guest Materials), P.O. Box 486, Weimar, CA, 95736. 1986.

Chapter 5

1. Keys, A., N. Kimura, A. Kusukawa, B. Bronte-Stewart, N. Larsen, and M. H. Keys: Lessons from the serum cholesterol studies in Japan, Hawaii, and Los Angeles. Ann Inter Med 48:83, 1958.
2. *Time*, March 26, 1984, 58–63.

Chapter 6

1. Biological Sciences, April 28, 1973.
2. Lutz, J., H. M. Linswiler, Am. J. Clin. Nutr. 34:2178–86, 1981.
3. Craig, Winstaron J. Ph.D., M.P.H., R.D., "Calcium Losses Caused by High Protein Diets," *Health & Healing*, Spring, 1983, 12–13.
4. Clark, Matt, et al, "The Calcium Craze." *Newsweek*. January 27, 1986, 48–52.
5. Mazess, R. B. *American Journal of Clinical Nutrition*. 27:916, 1974.
6. Draper, H. H. and R. R. Bell. Adv. Nutr. Res. 2:79–106, 1979.
7. Marsh, A. G., T. V. Sanches, O. Mickelsen, et al. *Journal of the American Diet Association*, 76:148–151, 1980.
8. Hegsted, M. and H. M. Linkswiler. Journal of Nutrition 11:244–51, 1981.
9. Brenner, B. M., T. W. Meyer, T. H. Hostetter. New England Journal of Medicine. 307:652–9, 1982.
10. Robertson, W. G., P. J. Heyburn, M. Peacock, et al. Clin. Sci. 57:285–8, 1979.
11. Wohl and Goodhart, *Modern Nutrition in Health and Disease*, 4th ed., Lea & Febiger, Philadelphia, 1968.
12. Linkswiler, H. M., M. B. Zemel, H. Hegsted, et al. Fed. Proc. 40:2429–33, 1981.
13. Allen, L. H., E. A. Oddoye, S. Margen. *American Journal of Clinical Nutrition*. 32:741–9, 1979.
14. R. Bressani and M. Behar. *The Use of Plant Protein Foods in Preventing*

Malnutrition. Proceedings of the Sixth International Congress of Nutrition. Edinburgh. August 9–15, 1963. Edinburgh, E & S. Livingston, Ltd., 1964. M. G. Hardinge, H. Crooks, and F. Stare. Nutritional studies of vegetarians. 5. Proteins and essential amino acids. *J. Am. Dietet. Ac.* 48:25. 1966. M. Sahyun, ed. *Proteins and Amino Acids in Nutrition.* New York, Reinhold Publishing Corp., 1948. A. Sanchez, J. A. Scharffenberg, and U. D. Register. Nutritive value of selected proteins and protein combinations. 1. The biological value of proteins singly and in meal patterns with varying fat composition. *Am. J. Clin. Nutrition* 13:243, 1963. D. M. Hegsted, V. Kent, A. G. Tsongas, and F. J. Stare. A comparison of the nutritive value of proteins in mixed diets for dogs, rats, and human beings. *J. Lab. & Clin. Med.* 32:403, 1947. D. M. Hegsted, M. F. Trulson, and H. S. White. Lysine and methionine supplementation of all-vegetable diets for human adults. *J. Nutrition.* 56:555, 1955.

Chapter 7
1. Milton G. Crane, M.D. "Does 'Everybody' Need Milk?" *Weimar Bulletin* Vol. 9 No. 3. April, May 1985.
2. R. S. Moore. *The China Doctor.* Harper & Row. 1960.
3. Frank A. Oski, M.D. *Don't Drink Your Milk!.* Mollica Press, Ltd, Syracuse, N.Y. 1983, 24.
4. Ibid. 14–15.
5. Oski, Ibid.
6. Crane, Ibid.
7. Mollica Press, Ltd, New York, 1983.
8. Crane, Ibid.
9. Walker & Isselbach. Ibid.
10. Gerard, J. W., Mackenzie, J. W. A., Goluboff, N., et al: "Cow's Milk Allergy; Prevalence and Manifestations in an Unselected Series of Newborns." *Acta Paediatr Scand,* Supplement 234, 1973.
11. Fleming, D. W. S. L. Cochi, K. L. MacDonald, et al: "Pasteurized Milk as a Vehicle of Infection in an Outbreak of Listerosis," *New England Journal of Medicine,* 312:404–407, 1985.
12. Oski, Ibid. 32–33.
13. C. Olson, L. S. Miller, et al: "Transmission of lymphosarcoma from cattle to sheep." *J. Nat. Cancer Institute.* 49:1463, 1972. H. M. McClure, M. E. Keeling, R. P. Cluster, et al: "Erythroleukemia in two infant champanzees fed milk from cows naturally infected with bovine C-type virus." *Cancer Research.* 34: 2745–57, 1974.
14. Crane, ibid.
15. Mervyn Hardinge, M.D., D.P.H., Ph.D. (Pharmacology), "Cheese and Cheese Products." REVIEW & HERALD, 24 Oct. 1974, 12–13.
16. Ibid.
17. U.S. Department of Agriculture, *Cheese Varieties and Descriptions.* Agriculture Handbook No. 54. 1953.
18. M. S. Jarvik, L. S. Goodman and A. Gilman, *The Pharmaceutical Basis of Therapeutics,* New York, The Macmillan Company, 1970. 185.
19. Leon Unger, M.D., and Joel L. Cristol, M.D. "Allergic Migraine." *Annals of Allergy* 28:106–109. March 1970.

Chapter 8
1. H. A. Harper, et. al.; Review of Physiological Chemistry, 16th ed., Lange Medical Publication. 1977, 401., Los Altos, CA.
2. Genesis 9; Leviticus 17.
3. Leviticus 11 and 17.
4. Psalm 90:10.
5. Virginia Morell, "Fishing for Trouble," and Russ Rymer, "America's Fish: Safe to Eat?" *International Wildlife*, July–August 1984. 40–43.
6. Ibid.
7. Ibid.
8. Ibid.
9. *Statistical Summary Federal Meat and Poultry Inspection for Fiscal Year 1984.* USDA Bulletin FSIS–14, April 1985.
10. Owen S. Parrett, M.D. "Why I Don't Eat Meat," (Reprint) *Life and Health*, Washington, D.C. 20012.
11. 4:1, March 1986.
12. LLU Data
13. Personal Letter to Raymond Moore, Nov. 20, 1973, 83 Stevenson Street, San Francisco, CA 94105.
14. *Farmers Bulletin* No. 1069, 4.
15. *Consumer Reports*, August 1971, 478.
16. *The Ministry*, November 1976.
17. O. Gregor, R. Toman, and F. Prusova, "Gastrointestinal Cancer and Nutrition." *Gut* 10:1031–1034, 1969; *Newsweek*, Feb. 18, 1974, 80, 83.
18. D. Schottenfeld, *Cancer Epidemiology and Prevention, Current Concepts,* (Springfield, Ill: Charles C. Thomas, 1975), 574.
19. C. H. Best and N. B. Taylor, *The Physiological Basis of Medical Practice,* 6th ed. (Baltimore: The Williams and Wilkins Company, 1955), 102.
20. J. R. Cooper, F. E. Bloom, and R. H. Roth, *The Biochemical Basis of Neuropharmacology,* 2nd ed. (New York: Oxford University Press, 1974), 14.

Chapter 9
1. University of California, Berkeley, *Wellness Letter*, 2:7. April 1986.
2. Baldwin, B. E., and M. V. Baldwin, Effects of Some Flavor Chemicals on Electrical Activity of Gastric Vagus, Brain, Heart and Integrity of Gastric Mucosa. Proc. Inter. Union of Physiol. Sciences, XIII:47 (1977).
3. Marjorie V. Baldwin, M.D., and Bernell E. Baldwin, Ph.D. "SPICES—Recipe for Trouble." *Wildwood Echoes*, Winter 1978–79.
4. A. Osol, G. E. Farrar, Jr., K. H. Beyer, Jr., D. K. Detweiler, J. H. Brown, Robertson Pratt, H. W. Youngken; The Dispensatory of the United States of America, 25th edition. (Philadelphia: J.B. Lippincott Co. 1960) 328, 333, 335–337: "Cinnamon. N.F.," "Ceylon Cinnamon," "Cinnamon Oil" and "Clove," respectively.
5. H. W. Davenport, Physiology of the Digestive Tract, 3rd edition (Chicago: Year Book Medical Publishers, Inc., 1971) 117. And F. Hollander and R. L. Goldfischer, *Journal of the National Cancer Institute*, 10:339–354, 1949–1950.
6. A. Osol, et al, op. cit.
7. J. Levy and E. Michel-Ber, "Ganglion-exciting effects of increasing doses

of nicotine on the isolated eserinized duodenum of the rat." Compt. Rend. Soc. Biol. 148, 1539–41 (1954) 1955.

8. F. Hollander, F. U. Lauber and J. Stein. "Some characteristics of gastric secretion induced by mustard oil suspension." Am. J. Physiol. 148, 724–31 (1947), 5983.

9. *Tufts University Diet & Nutrition Letter*. Vol. 4, No. 3. May 1986.

10. Vol. 2, No. 2. November 1985.

11. *Nutrition Reviews*, Vol. 38, 274–275, 1980.

12. F. A. Vorhes and F. J. Lehman, "New Problems of Food Safety," Public Health Reports, Vol. 71, 571–576, 1956.

13. Brooks and Lucy Fuller, *Whole Foods for Whole People*. 3rd Ed., P.O. Box 701, Webster, FL 33597, 12–3.

14. Ibid.

Chapter 11

1. Kellock, Brian. *The Fiber Man*, Lion Publishing Corporation, Michigan, 1985. 183.

2. K. O'Dea, P. J. Nestel, L. Antonoff, in *Am. J. Clin. Nutr.*, 33:760–765, 1980.

3. G. B. Haber, K. W. Heaton, D. Murphy, in *Lancet*, 2:679–682, 1977.

4. G. H. Joseph, *Nutrition Research*, Sept, 1955.

5. *J. of Am. Med. Assoc.*, Nov. 18, 1961.

6. Haynes, Tompkins, Washburn, Winteres *Society of Experimental Biology and Medical Proceedings* back in 1937.

7. See also Denis P. Burkitt, M.D., F.R.C.S, "Dietary Fiber and Cancers of the Western World." From keynote lecture at the second annual Bristol-Myers Symposium on Nutrition Research. Washington, D.C., December 9–10, 1982. Published in *Health and Healing*, Spring 1983.

8. 2 Kings 5.

Chapter 12

1. 1 Corinthians 10:31.

2. *Tufts University Diet and Nutrition Letter*. 2:8. October 1984.

3. Ibid., Vol. 1, No. 10, Dec. 1983.

4. Ibid. 2:8. Oct. 1985.

5. Ibid., Vol. 2, No. 2 "Measuring your life with coffee spoons." April 1984.

6. Ibid., Vol. 1, No. 6 "Caffeine reimplicated in heart disease." August 1983. Also April 1984 and October 1984.

7. Ibid., Vol. 2, No. 2. "Measuring your life with coffee spoons." April 1984. And "The spotlight is on caffeine again." Vol. 2, No. 2, October 1984.

8. Ibid., Special Report. "Herbal Teas Pack a Wallop.

9. Vol. 2, No. 4, January 1986.

10. Varro Tyler, *The Honest Herbal*. George F. Stickley, Co. Philadelphia. Also Tufts University *Diet & Nutrition Letter*, Vol. 4, No. 4, June 1986, 7–8 (Nd). University of California, Berkeley WELLNESS LETTER. Vol. 2, No. 4, January 1986. 8.

11. W. R. Kreiser and R. A. Martin, *J. Assoc. Off. Analy. Chem.* 61(6), 1978. Further information is available from KIRK-OTHMER: ENCYCLOPEDIA

OF CHEMICAL TECHNOLOGY, Vol. 6, Third Ed., John Wiley & Sons, Inc. 1979.

12. J. W. McFarland, M.D. "The Real Fountain of Youth," *Life & Health*, July 1981.

13. M. G. Hardinge, M.D. "Water, Water, Water." Film by Loma Linda University School of Health, Loma Linda, CA. 1972.

Chapter 13

1. Luce, Gay Gaer; *Biological Rhythms in Human and Animal Physiology*, Dover Publications Inc., N.Y., 1971.

2. *American Health*, November, 1984, 66.

3. Siegel, P. V., Gerathewol, S. J., and Mohler, S. R. "Time-Zone Effects," *Science*, 1969, 164, 1249–ff.

4. Raymond S. Moore, *China Doctor*. Harper & Row, New York. 1960.

5. Moore, ibid, 115.

6. Isaiah 26:3.

7. Mark 6:31, LB.

8. Ecclesiastes 3:1.

Chapter 14

1. Arthur Guyton, M.D., *Textbook of Medical Physiology, 4th Ed..* W. B. Saunders Co. Philadelphia. 1971. 863.

2. Ullensvand, L. P. Thirty percent of food intake is by snacking. Food consumption patterns in the seventies. *Vital Speeches of the Day* 36:240, Feb. 1, 1970.

3. Lynch, M., "Between-Meal Snacks," *Signs of the Times*, June 1978, 22.

4. Cereal Institute Inc., *Breakfast Source Book*, Chicago, IL.

5. Bud Getchell, Ph.D., *Being Fit: A Personal Guide*. John Wiley & Sons, 605 Third Ave., New York 10016.

6. Kenneth Cooper, M.D. *The New Aerobics*. M. Evans, distributed in association with Lippincott, 1970.

Chapter 15

1. Dobson, James. *The Struggle with Obesity: The Overweight Woman*. Focus on the Family tape CS218, Arcadia, CA 91006. 1982.

Chapter 16

1. Richard A. Hansen, "Healing Sunlight," *Health and Healing*, Summer, 1982.

2. Zane Kime, M.D. *Sunlight*. World Health Publications, Box 400, Penryn, CA 95663. p. 27.

Chapter 17

1. Crowther, J. A. *Ions, Electrons and Ionizing Radiations*. Edward Arnold and Company. London 1938.

2. Windischbauer, A. *Die Naturlichen Heilkraefte von Bad-Gastein*. Springer Verlag. Wien 1958.

3. Martin, T. L., Jr. *Climate Control Through Ionization*. J Franklin Institute. 254:267–280, 1952.

4. Krueger, A. P. ~*Air Ions and Physiological Function.* The Journal of General Physiology. 45:1962. 233–241. Also study by Doctors Jordan and Lakeland, reported in *EEG,* Eastern Association. 1957.

5. Kjeldsen, K. P., Astrup and J. Wanstrup. "Reversal of Rabbit Atheromatosis by Hyperoxia." *Journal of Atherosclerosis Research.* 10:173. 1969.

6. Swank, R. and Cullen, C. F. *Circulatory Changes in the Hamster's Cheek Pouch Associated with Alimentary Lipemia.* Proceedings of the Society of Experimental and Biological Medicine. 82:381. 1953. Also Friedman, M. and Rosenman, R. *Circulation XXIX.* 874. 1974.

7. Chen, George, *Put Air to Work for You.* Weimar Bulletin. 3:4, April 1979.

Chapter 18

1. Luke 8:22–25; Proverbs 3:6.

2. David M. Rorvik, "How Diet Can Affect Your Mind," *McCalls,* April 1972. p. 39.

3. Isaiah 26:3.

4. Philippians 3:20, NIV.

5. 1 Peter 2:9.

6. Romans 8:14–17.

7. Revelation 3:20–21.

8. Exodus 20:12.

9. Matthew 5,6,7.

10. Matthew 7:12.

11. William Wilson, M.D. "The Therapy of Prayer," *Guideposts.* July 1978.

12. Ephesians 4:26.

13. Warren Peters, M.D. "Stress and Cancer." Unpublished paper, Hartland Institute, Rapidan, VA. 1986.

14. 1 John 4:18.

15. J. Lynch, *The Broken Heart: The Medical Consequences of Loneliness.* Basic Books, N.Y. 1979, 44.

16. A. Kraus. "Some Epidemiologic Aspects of the High Mortality Rate in the Young Widowed Group." *Journ. Chr. Dis. 10:207–217. 1959.*

17. Peters, ibid.

18. *Ibid.*

19. Matthew 6:12.

Chapter 19

1. *Woman's Day.* April, 1985. 170.

2. *Family Circle,* October, 1985, 72–76.

3. *Tufts University Diet and Nutrition Letter,* Vol. 1, No. 10, Dec. 1983.

4. *Tufts University Diet and Nutrition Letter,* Vol. 1, No. 3, May 1983.

5. *The Children's Health Connection,* Vol. 3, No. 3, Dec. 1984.

6. Martin Engel, "Rapunzel, Rapunzel, Let Down Your Golden Hair: Some Thoughts on Early Childhood Education." Unpublished manuscript. U.S. Office of Education, Washington, D.C., about 1975.

7. John Bowlby, *Maternal Care and Mental Health,* Geneva: World Health

Organization, 1952. See also the authors' books: *Better Late Than Early, Home Grown Kids, Home Spun Schools, Home Style Teaching, School Can Wait,* and their Columbia University Teacher's College Record monograph, "Research and Common Sense," Winter 1982–83.

8. U. Bronfenbrenner, *Two Worlds of Childhood.* New York, Simon and Schuster, 1970. 102.

Chapter 20

1. Tufts University *Diet and Nutrition Letter* 3:10, December, 1985, "Special Report."

Chapter 21

1. Goldstein, Clifford, *Health and Healing,* Fall, 1982. 14.
2. Ex. 16:3; Num. 11:4,5.
3. Job 10:10; Ex. 3:8 and Deut. 32:14.
4. Crane, Milton G., "Diseases of the Egyptians and God's Answer to Them," Unpublished paper. Weimar Institute, Weimar, CA. 1984.
5. 1 Cor. 10:31; 6:19, and Rom. 12:1,2.
6. Gen. 1:26, 27.
7. John 14:6.
8. John 5:6; 7:23; Acts 9:34; Phil. 2:5.
9. Phil. 2:5.

INDEX